Needs Assessment and Community Care:
Clinical Practice and Policy Making

Needs Assessment and Community Care: Clinical Practice and Policy Making

Edited by

Steve Baldwin DipTech BAHons MSc Dip Clin Psychol PhD

Associate Professor
Faculty of Health and Human Sciences
Edith Cowan University
Western Australia

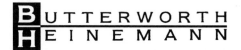

BUTTERWORTH
HEINEMANN

Butterworth-Heinemann
Linacre House, Jordan Hill, Oxford OX2 8DP
225 Wildwood Avenue, Woburn, MA 01801-2041
A division of Reed Educational and Professional Publishing Ltd

A member of the Reed Elsevier plc group

OXFORD   BOSTON   JOHANNESBURG
MELBOURNE   NEW DELHI   SINGAPORE

First published 1998

© Reed Educational and Professional Publishing Ltd 1998

British Library Cataloguing in Publication Data
A catalogue record for this book is available from the British Library

Library of Congress Cataloguing in Publication Data
A catalogue record for this book is available from the Library of Congress

ISBN 0 7506 2435 3

Typeset by Bath Typesetting, Bath
Printed and bound in Great Britain by Biddles Ltd, Guildford and King's Lynn

Contents

List of contributors   vii
Preface   ix
Acknowledgements   xiii

1 Problems with needs: where theory meets practice in
    mental health services   1
    Steve Baldwin

2 Assessing health care need: the conceptual foundation   9
    Per-Erik Liss

3 Assessment of need and case management: an evolving
    concept   25
    Peter A. Woods, Steve Baldwin

4 Needs assessment in a rehabilitation service   43
    Karen Black

5 Assessing the needs of people who are disabled by serious
    ongoing mental health problems   55
    Julie Repper, Rachel Perkins

6 Needs assessment in elderly people suffering from
    communication difficulties and/or cognitive impairment   73
    Ingalill Rahm Hallberg

7 The antinomies of choice in community care   89
    Kirsten Stalker

8 Feminist perspectives on community care in Australia   99
    Melanie Edwards

9 Aspects of informal care in Northern Ireland   113
    Eileen Evason

10 Co-creation of pathology: when psychological factors are
    secondary to socioeconomic factors   124
    Christine Meier, Giorgio Rezzonico

11 Psychosocial intervention in nursing: a structural model
    for holistic care   140
    Gloria Novel

12 Slovene mental health services   151
    David Brandon, Vito Flaker

13   Care of people with chronic mental disorders:
     a European–American perspective   161
     John Talbott
14   Producing irreversible change: the process of transforming
     an old-fashioned hospital into a modern treatment centre   169
     Fanny Duckert
15   Survivor-led research in human services: challenging the
     dominant medical paradigm   186
     Jan Wallcraft
16   Assessing learning outcomes in post-qualifying
     community care training   209
     Jane Shears, Shula Ramon, Edna Conlon

Index   219

Contributors

Steve Baldwin DipTech, BA(Hons), MSc, Dip Clin Psychol, PhD
Associate Professor, Department of Psychology, Edith Cowan
University, Bunbury, Western Australia

Karen Black BSc
Research Psychologist, Airedale NHS Trust, Moor Lane Centre,
Burley-in-Wharfedale, West Yorkshire

David Brandon
Professor in Community Care, Anglia Polytechnic University,
Cambridge

Edna Conlon PhD
Chairperson, UKAN, Sheffield

Fanny Duckert PhD
Professor, Institute of Psychology, University of Oslo, Oslo, Norway

Melanie Edwards BA
Voluntary Community Worker, Women's Community Centre, Stepney,
South Australia

Eileen Evason BA, MSc
Professor in Social Administration and Policy, University of Ulster,
Northern Ireland

Vito Flaker PhD
Lecturer in Social Work, University of Ljubijana, Slovenia

Ingalill Rahm Hallberg PhD
Professor in Caring Sciences, Lund University, Lund, Sweden

Per-Erik Liss PhD
Associate Professor, Department of Health and Society, Linkoping University, Linkoping, Sweden

Christine Meier PhD
Director, Centro al Dragonato, Bellinzona, Ticino, Switzerland; and Visiting Professor, University of Milan, Milan, Italy

Gloria Novel PhD
Director of Master of Mental Health Nursing, School of Nursing, University of Barcelona, Barcelona, Spain

Rachel Perkins BA, MPhil, PhD
Clinical Director and Consultant Clinical Psychologist, Pathfinder Mental Health Services NHS Trust, Springfield University Hospital, London

Shula Ramon PhD
Professor of Health and Social Studies, Faculty of Health and Social Work, Anglia Polytechnic University, Cambridge

Julie Repper MPhil, BA(Hons), RMN, RGN
Research Fellow, Sheffield Centre for Health and Related Research, University of Sheffield, Sheffield

Giorgio Rezzonico MD
Associate Professor in Cognitive Psychology, Institute of Medical Psychology, University of Milan, Italy

Jane Shears
Researcher, Anglia Polytechnic University, Cambridge

Kirsten Stalker BA, CQSW, PhD
Senior Research Fellow, Social Work Research Centre, University of Stirling, Stirling

John Talbott MD
Professor and Chairman, University of Maryland, Baltimore; Director, Institute of Psychiatry and Human Behavior, Baltimore, USA

Jan Wallcraft, BSc(Hons)
Research Scholar, South Bank University, London

Peter A. Woods PhD, ABPsS
General Manager, Learning Disability Services, Gwynedd Community Health Trust, Ysbyty Bryn-y-Neuadd, Llanfairfechan, Gwynedd, Wales

Preface

During the 1980s, many human services practitioners and providers became highly dissatisfied with traditional problem-based approaches to service planning and provision. In health and social services, there was ongoing disenchantment with the orthodox models of delivery, based on conventional biomedical service templates.

The search for credible and practical alternatives to existing service models continued into the 1990s, without ultimate resolution of the ongoing debate. This text is aimed to provide a summary of some of the successful attempts to establish alternative services.

The development of 'needs assessment' and 'needs-based services' can be traced back to attempts by some service staff to establish alternative provision frameworks. Nonetheless in mental health services there has been considerable disagreement about the measurement of 'need'. Service planning, based on accurate identification of clients' real needs, has been restricted, due to poor conceptualization and weak methodologies. These core themes are explored in detail in the first chapter. These themes are revisited by Per-Erik Liss, in Chapter 2. He provides a clear exposition of the conceptual foundation about measurement of health care need, from a European perspective. In the third chapter, Peter Woods provides an incisive account of the interrelationship between needs assessment and case management approaches. The central thesis is that these two methods of data collection/recording are compatible, and can easily be accommodated together within the same service system.

Karen Black provides an overview of one successful UK attempt to locate needs assessment in a service setting. Her report provides a high level of detailed analysis which illuminates the process of transition to a needs-based service delivery system. In the subsequent chapter, Julie Repper and Rachel Perkins describe needs assessment with people who have serious mental health problems. This detailed account provides another commentary about process themes, based on implementation of a UK project. From a Scandinavian perspective, Ingalill Hallberg applies the concept of needs assessment to the specific population of elderly people. The special challenges associated with service provision for people with communication problems are outlined, with recommendations for future provision.

In the remaining chapters, generic, global themes associated with provision are explored in greater detail. In particular, the relevance and appropriateness of 'community care' concepts is examined, in the context of alternative service provision models.

Kirsten Stalker examines the concept of choice and provides a commentary about ways in which alternatives can be inbuilt into service structures. From Australia, Melanie Edwards provides an overview of feminist perspectives on 'community care' including an examination of some of the service rhetoric. In the next chapter, Eileen Evason offers data from a unique series of studies completed in Northern Ireland. Many of her conclusions will challenge orthodox views about service provision in this special cultural and political context.

Many detractors of alternative service provision models assert '. . . but it could never work in the *real* world . . .'. Christine Meier and Giorgio Rezzonico provide a detailed account of a European model from Ticino, Switzerland established to provide services for people with chronic mental health problems. Their work demonstrates successful long-term outcomes with a particularly challenging population. From Barcelona, Gloria Novel demonstrates how a psychosocial approach can be incorporated into an holistic model of care. Also from Europe, David Brandon and Vito Flaker provide an account about attempts to establish high quality services in Slovenia. In the era of considerable social and political reforms, their commentary generates an incisive critique.

With the benefit of an external perspective, John Talbott gives an account of deinstitutionalization attempts in the USA, compared with western European experiences. This powerful analysis will benefit practitioners, planners and researchers seeking a cross-cultural analysis.

Although many practitioners aspire to permanency in change attempts, few transformations achieve that outcome. From Norway, Fanny Duckert provides one account of irreversible change from traditional to non-traditional service provision. With a similar perspective, Jan Wallcraft provides a major challenge to the medical and psychiatric orthodoxy in mental health service provision. She rightly asserts the need for strong citizen and client advocacy. The text is concluded with a timely reminder by Jane Shears, Shula Ramon and Edna Conlon about the need for training agendas in mental health services. They provide an overview of an innovative UK training initiative.

This text is aimed to provide a bridge between theory and practice. The field of needs and needs assessment contains a sparse literature, based on a puny analysis of published material. With a cross-cultural and international focus, the text will be of interest to theoreticians, practitioners and researchers. In particular, the book will integrate contributions from different cultures and national perspectives, with a focus on integration and analysis.

The field of human services has reached a conceptual crossroads about patterns of service delivery. There is an unresolved need for integration of user perspectives. Services directed to meet individual need are also required, especially in the reconstructed purchaser-provider climate. Needs assessment and needs-led services provide a robust framework for future provision.

Steve Baldwin

Acknowledgements

Many thanks to Susan Devlin for her persistence and determination throughout this project. Thanks are due to Narelle Mattaboni for assistance with the preparation of the manuscript.

Chapter 1

Problems with needs: where theory meets practice in mental health services

Steve Baldwin

Introduction

Since the late 1970s there have been more efforts to integrate the assessment of 'needs' of people with mental health problems. Problem-based services have been rejected in favour of a 'needs-based' approach to planning and provision. Service design based on 'deficit' and 'defect' approaches have been viewed as contextually inappropriate to the true needs of people with mental health disorders. Practitioners often have been at the cutting edge of attempts to provide services according to need. In the mental health field, practitioners have borrowed concepts and ideas from other areas, including intellectual disability and physical disability. Generally, however, these attempts have been unplanned and not theory-driven nor based on empirical methods. Rather, practitioners in different agencies and organizations have developed their own patterns for provision. Examination of the 'needs assessment' literature reveals an ill-defined territory with a wide array of meanings and definitions. Some ways forward are identified, together with suggestions for improved practice.

Background history

Murray (1938) provided the definitive list of human needs to account for behaviour and motivation. The original list provided by Murray included needs connected to inanimate objects, expression of ambition, power, injury to self or others, affection and other social goals (e.g. play). This early attempt to specify the full range of human needs proved highly influential. In a later formulation, Maslow (1954) specified five different levels of need to describe the sequential and developmental nature of motivation in people. The psychological development of people was believed to relate to areas of physiological, safety, love, esteem and self-actualization needs.

The work of Murray and Maslow has been highly influential in the conceptualizations of needs and needs assessment. However, neither framework has been applied directly to working with people who have mental health problems. Contemporary approaches to needs assessment generally have included the related areas of health, employment, residence, mobility, education and leisure/recreation (e.g. Harding, Baldwin and Baser, 1986).

Other human service fields

In the field of intellectual disability there has been much discussion about needs-based service provision for clients. The concept has been integrated into planning and provision documents at local, regional and national levels in North America, Australia and the UK. Previously 'needs assessment' has been used to plan future services. Regrettably, however, there has been disparity among practitioners about the meanings of 'needs' and 'needs assessment' concepts. This uncertainty has extended into the area of intellectual conceptualizations about needs (e.g. Burton, 1990; Doyal and Gough, 1991; Pickin and St Leger, 1993).

Previously there has been considerable debate about the utility and validity of the concepts of needs and needs assessment (e.g. Horton, Corcoran and Anderson, 1975; Grossman, Kriklewicz and Chamberlain, 1976; Horton and Carr, 1976; Kimmel, 1977; Varenais, 1977). Recurrent problems have endured in the field, including: poorly applied assessment methodologies; ill-defined or unspecified needs; identified needs unmatched with existing services; poor descriptions of the client group (Lareau and Heumann, 1982). Also, many service planning and strategic planning documents have not provided a comprehensive analysis of the range of client needs. Often, provision agencies have merely replicated existing service templates, excluding consideration of special needs services. Specifically, '... typical needs assessments may be counterproductive, resulting in misleading or incorrect findings...' (Lareau and Heumann, 1982). There is no uniform definition of needs assessment, with a wide variation between services and practitioners.

Definitions, validity and utility

One core problem of the needs assessment field has been the multiple use of the term in different settings. The term has been used to 'explain' both 'needs for services' (Goodman and Craig, 1982) and 'needs of individual clients with a mental health problem' (Lareau, 1983). According to the first definition, needs assessments have been used as a device to measure epidemiological demand; existing service usage has been used to calculate future service demands. These two different approaches have produced dissimilar templates of service provision. Services planned and provided around the individual needs of consumers and clients will allow planners and providers to create more personalized, flexible and idiosyncratic responses to need.

The concept of needs assessment has also been used to provide staff training and resource management planning (Newstrom and Lilyquist, 1979; Steadham, 1980). In occupational therapy services, needs assessment has been used to establish educational, planning, training and organizational goals (Bullard, 1983). The defined needs assessment model included both pre-assessment data collection and reporting back about findings. Using this perspective, needs assessment is used to define the activities of staff in the service. Training or educational goals are identified to determine behavioural changes. Such an approach is based on involvement at the second (staff) or third (system) level, rather than at the first (client) level. This use of needs assessment is distinct from the traditional approach, which is explicitly focused on a primary level involvement with clients.

Another usage of needs assessment has been in the field of physical disability. The use of questionnaire data has been employed as an audit device to collect information about the identified needs of clients with a physical disability, including stated needs and unresolved problems (Omohundro *et al.*, 1983). Data were collated about income level, employment, health and use of existing services. Specific areas of concern were identified by clients, including physical and emotional problems, housework completion, unresolved employment problems and limits on mobility. Service provision agencies had not resolved these problems; clients often did not use existing services, as they did not know of their existence. Improved service provision for these clients with a physical disability would have required more flexible, localized services.

Range of needs assessment methods

The diverse range of meanings of needs and needs assessment has prevented clarity in the field of mental health services. One definition has exerted considerable influence since the 1970s (Bradshaw, 1972). According to Bradshaw, four different definitions of need were possible: (i) normative need, a desirable standard to measure existing services if differences existed, needs were identified; (ii) felt need, perceived needs, or 'what people really want' (although people do not always know what is in their best interest and limited knowledge about options may restrict their choices); (iii) expressed need, a felt need shifted into action, a stated demand for services, a felt need acted on by that person; and (iv) comparative need, identified by people already receiving that service, if other similar people do not currently receive that service they are 'in need'. Some similarity between the approaches of (i) and (ii) exists whereby 'experts' are actively involved in the prescription of services on behalf of clients.

The concept of needs assessment has also been subject to multiple interpretations, definitions and attached meanings. In 1983, Bullard identified three different types of needs assessment, including (i) survey, (ii) audit and (iii) interview methods. Lareau (1983) identified five different methods of needs assessments, including (i) survey, (ii) secondary data use, (iii) key informant, (iv) group process/public hearings and (v) service use statistics. Each of these five methods produced dissimilar outcomes about the type and range of services identified. It was evident that the nature and type of source data exerted considerable influence on the quality of services received by client groups.

Problems of use of needs and needs assessment in mental health settings

There is no shared single understanding of either needs or needs assessment in mental health service settings; both planners and practitioners have used the terms without adequate definition and precision. In the field of intellectual disability this terminological confusion has been especially damaging. Many clients with an intellectual impairment have not been able to express their own needs assertively. Preferences between service options have been particularly difficult to assess accurately with this client population. Service planning and provision with this client group has produced multiple tensions between professionals, family members and clients.

In the context of this confusion, one commentator has recommended that the term 'needs' be abandoned (Williams, 1978). Support for this radical position has been marshalled from the observation that the terms 'needs' and 'needs assessment' have been used uncritically and indiscriminately across service settings. This lack of clarity has occurred due to: (i) lack of interdisciplinary service planning/provision, and (ii) absence of any sound theory for needs (Taylor-Gooby and Dale, 1981) or needs assessment (Lareau, 1983). Moreover '... needs assessment is considered by experts to be an essential part of mental health planning. Unfortunately, almost anything can pass for a needs assessment...' (Royse and Drude, 1982).

Needs assessments should be completed to assist clients. Unfortunately, the needs assessment process can be distorted to meet service requirements, rather than the true needs of consumers/clients. Inadequate, incomplete or inelegant needs assessments will produce misleading and inappropriate patterns of provision. Such distorted patterns will not assist client growth and development. In the field of intellectual disability it is essential to have a specified full range of generic and special needs services. The planning of adequate services for clients with an intellectual disability requires an explicit method to specify comprehensive and precise patterns of provision for individual clients. Previously, inadequate or puny forms of needs assessment have been used to ration the delivery of service provision. Staff who work in the area of needs assessment should develop a commitment to excellence in provision.

The potential for a conflict of interest between client and service needs has been identified. In the extreme, professional interests may dominate the ways in which services have been specified: '... a programme is justified by reference to the needs of the individual or needs of the community which the programme is meant to satisfy...' (Lawson, 1975).

Moreover, the service focus on 'meeting needs' can be inappropriate if client interests are deflected in favour of service priorities. The professional territorialization of 'needs' has been well documented. Human service professionals often determine the needs of clients, sometimes to meet their own interests. This conflict of interests has been identified (Illich, 1977; McKnight, 1977; Wiltshire, 1983). The province of needs assessment has been liable to the interests of health professionals. Territorialization of the field has been a real concern during the 1990s.

In the field of medicine, physicians have tended to use epidemiological methods to determine service provision for people with mental health problems. In contrast, non-medical specialists have favoured the use of needs assessment methods to determine subsequent provision. Such non-medical staff have thus expanded their province via the use of individual assessment techniques. In the field of intellectual disability, staff who complete needs assessment procedures also have used advocacy services to assist with separation of function between providers and clients. The relative independence of advocates has been especially useful in the completion of needs assessment methods.

Despite the attractions associated with needs-based service provision, there is no objective reality or absolute scale by which needs can be determined. Statements about needs are value-judgements, which reflect the beliefs and behaviours of the observer, based on ideas about the 'good life' (Bradshaw, 1972; Lawson, 1975). The contrasting proposition is that 'service use' statistics can be used to determine need levels; this assertion, however, should be challenged, as such measures can only reflect existing service usage. Moreover, such techniques continue to locate the problem or the source of the deficit within the person. Ideally, individual clients should remain at the core of service design and planning. Service planning based on estimates of groups of clients are spurious as a barometer of true need levels. It is politically unsound to continue to plan and provide mental health services around the identified needs of groups of clients.

Practical implications

The focus on an individual framing of client problems has set the conditions whereby professional interests have been enhanced. Even the contemporary focus on needs assessment has encouraged staff to professionalize their activities. The ability to state needs accurately suggests indispensability, expertise and high-level professional activity. The power to define people as clients has been viewed as a core hallmark activity of the health professional (Illich, 1977). High-tech language about the activities of professionals should not produce barriers to the active participation of people with a mental health problem.

The increased involvement of people with a mental health problem in service provision is a core concept associated with needs assessment and needs-based services. There are many unresolved tensions associated with traditional problem-based services. Failure to specify accurately the core activities of needs assessment may risk under-provision and the inappropriate delivery of services to clients. Practitioners should develop a more sophisticated awareness of their powerful role in service planning and provision. The trend toward multi-level needs assessment (Baldwin *et al.*, 1990) is one example of this improved understanding of political aspects of provision. Such methods make simultaneous statements about the desirable and necessary changes required by both staff and clients, within the context of the wider service system. This focus on the provision environment as well as the client may assist resource management (Harding, Baldwin and Baser, 1986).

Conclusions

Failure to specify accurately the twin concepts of needs and needs assessments risks devaluing of the process of service delivery for people with mental health problems. Clarity about these terms, and shared meaning among practitioners, should assist in the establishment of improved setting conditions for high-quality service provision.

References

Baldwin, S., Harding, K., Baser, C. (1990) *Multi-level needs assessment.* London: British Association of Behavioural Psychotherapy.

Bradshaw, J. (1972) The concept of social need. *New Society*, 19, 640–643.

Bullard, M. (1983) A needs assessment strategy for educational planning. *American Journal of Occupational Therapy*, 37, 624–629.

Burton, J. (1990) *Conflict: Human Needs Theory.* London: Macmillan.

Doyal, L., Gough, I. (1991) *A Theory of Human Need.* London: Macmillan.

Goodman, A. B., Craig, T. J. (1982) A needs assessment strategy for limited resources, *American Journal of Epidemiology*, 115, 624–632.

Grossman, M., Kriklewicz, E., Chamberlain, P. (1976) *A Comparative Assessment of Contemporary Procedures to Determine Housing Needs.* Lansing: Michigan State Housing Development Authority.

Harding, K., Baldwin, S., Baser, C. (1987) Towards multi-level needs assessments. *Behavioural Psychotherapy*, 15, 134–143.

Horton, G. T., Corcoran, G., Anderson, E. D. (1975) *Needs Assessment in a Title XX State Social Services Planning System*. Atlanta: Human Services Institute for Children and Families Incorporated.

Horton, G. T., Carr, V. M. E., (1976) *Techniques for Needs Assessments: State Experiences and Suggested Approaches to Title XX of the Social Security Act*. Washington, DC: Social and Rehabilitation Services, Public Service Administration Department of Health and Welfare.

Illich, I. (1977) *Disabling Professions*. London: Marion Boyars.

Kimmel, W. A. (1977) *Needs Assessment: A Critical Perspective*. Washington, DC: Office of Program Systems OAS for Planning and Evaluation, Department of Health, Education and Welfare.

Lareau, L. S. (1983) Needs assessments of the elderly: conclusions and methodological approaches. *The Gerontologist*, **23**, 518–526.

Lareau, L. S., Heumann, L. F. (1982) The inadequacy of needs assessments of the elderly. *The Gerontologist*, **22**, 324–330.

Lawson, K. (1975) *Philosophical Concepts and Values in Higher Education*. Nottingham: University of Nottingham/NIAE.

McKnight, J. (1977) Professionalised service and disabling help. In *Disabling Professions*. (I. Illich, ed.) London: Marion Boyars.

Maslow, A. H. (1954) *Motivation and Personality*. New York: Harper.

Murray, H. A. (1938) *Explorations in Personality*. New York: Oxford University Press.

Newstrom, J., Lilyquist, J. (1979) Selecting needs analysis methods. *Training and Development Journal*, **33**, 52–56.

Omohundro, J., Schneider, M. J., Marr, J. N., Grannermann, B. D. (1983) A four country needs assessment of rural disabled people. *Journal of Rehabilitation*, **49**, 19–24.

Pickin, C., St Leger, S. (1993) *Assessing Human Need Using the Life Cycle Framework*. Buckingham: Open University Press.

Royse, D., Drude, K. (1982) Mental health needs assessment: beware of false promises. *Community Mental Health Journal*, **18**, 97–106.

Steadham, S. (1980) Learning to select a needs assessment strategy. *Training and Development Journal*, **34**, 56–61.

Taylor-Gooby, P., Dale, J. (1981) *Social Theory and Social Welfare*. London: Edward Arnold.

Varenais, K. (1977) *Needs Assessment: an Explanatory Critique*. OAS for Planning and Education. Washington, DC: Department of Health, Education and Welfare.

Williams, A. (1978) Need – an economic exegesis. In *Economic Aspects of Health Services* (A. Culyer, K. Wright, eds). Oxford: Martin Robertson.

Wiltshire, H. (1983) The concepts of learning and need in adult education. *Studies in Adult Education*, **5**, 26–30.

Chapter 2
Assessing health care need: the conceptual foundation

Per-Erik Liss

Introduction

Discussions about needs are frequent in everyday life. The term need is often used to describe a certain context of people, and there are sometimes quarrels about needs. The reason for the central position of needs in the culture is that needs are related to human suffering. Needs normally indicate urgency. They indicate that something vital is missing. They therefore exercise a certain kind of force. When people care for their fellow human beings, they are typically sensitive to needs.

Needs also exercise force at the societal level. All societies that want to look after their members are interested in how the human needs are met, although they differ concerning the methods of meeting the needs (for instance, with respect to governmental intervention). Social policies therefore consider needs as something central, and health policies in particular are sensitive to needs. For instance, the Swedish Public Health Act lays down that the policies of the health care system shall be determined only by the needs of the individuals. Knowledge about the population's need for health care is central to such a policy, and the assessment of health care need will be a fundamental issue.

Several different methods or strategies are suggested for the assessment of health care need. They all have in common that they measure the need only indirectly, which creates some concern regarding the validity of the methods. The validity concerns the extent to which a method measures what it is supposed to measure. Take for example the indicator approach – to what extent does it measure the health care need?

This approach consists, roughly, of making inferences of needs from descriptive statistics. The basic premise of indicator analyses is that certain constellations of characteristics are related to health hazard, ill health or need of care. By measuring the indicators in a certain area it is possible to get a view of the area's status in respect of ill health or health hazard. Factors often discussed in this context include mortality, morbidity, age, sex, marital status, occupation and income. The factors can be combined into a formula. For instance the RAWP formula, used in the UK, was based on data about age, sex and mortality.

The inferences of health care needs in this type of strategy can be described in two stages: from information given by the indicators to a view of the health status of the population; from a view of health status to an opinion as to health care needs.

The validity of the first stage can of course be questioned. What picture of health status do the factors give? Is it, for instance, certain that age always is a valid measure of degree of health or ill health, or that it is occupation or income? However, the second stage is the more interesting here. To what extent does information about health status provide information about health care need? Is information about health status sufficient for the assessment of health care need?

This method involves some uncertainties concerning technical issues of measurement, but the fundamental uncertainty involved in the method is due to a deep-level defect. It is due to a lack of conceptual analysis. What is a need of health care? Is it sufficient to relate it vaguely to the population's state of ill health or the population's demand for health care?

The purpose of this chapter is to present some of the results of a philosophical investigation into the concept of health care need (Liss, 1993). This means first outlining the logical structure of the general concept of need. The most significant characteristic of this concept is the goal of need. Without a clear understanding of this goal it is pointless to claim that someone has a need. From this theoretical basis the concept of health care need is analysed.

It will be argued that health is a significant component of health care need and, drawing on a holistic theory of health, a teleological concept of health care need will be presented. The implications for the setting of priorities in accordance with health care need will be discussed, and finally the basic structure of a model for the assessment of health care need will be presented.

Concepts of need

In the literature on need (or concept of need) two different traditions can be discerned. In one, need is considered as a *tension* or a *disequilibrium* in the organism. A living organism strives to keep itself in balance. It is said to be struggling to maintain homeostasis. Disturbances, induced by internal or external stimuli, lead to tensions in the organism. The term 'need' is used to designate these tensions. This need can be called a *tension need*.

The tension or disequilibrium triggers off behaviours towards certain objects. Getting hold of these objects is expected to lead to reduction or elimination of the tension. Needs are satisfied when the tension is eliminated. What things people need can be determined, according to this view, by studying people's behaviour. The need for water is an example of a typical tension need. A person who suffers from shortage of body fluid and feels thirsty will become disposed to look for water.

In the second tradition need is considered as something instrumental or teleological. This need can be called a *teleological need*. The fact that there is a need, and what there is a need of, is here related to a certain goal. There is a need of food, for instance, in order to survive, and there is a need of love in order to live well. The statement 'P needs X if X is necessary for realizing a certain goal' illustrates this view. That a certain thing is necessary for realizing a goal implies that the thing is lacking: there is a deficiency of some kind. Or, to put it otherwise, there is a *gap* between what is and what should be. Assume a situation where it is said that Mr Smith has a need for a wheelchair. This locution is typically used when Mr Smith lacks the wheelchair (what is) and the wheelchair is necessary in order for Mr Smith to live a decent life (what should be).

According to the two views of need, the term need can be used to refer to two different things: either to a tension in the organism, or to a situation of lack (or a gap) related to a goal. The two views might in certain circumstances coincide. A person who suffers from, for instance, shortage of body fluid and feels thirsty might be said to have both a tension need and a teleological need for water.

It is important, however, to notice that the two views of need are fundamentally different. To assess human needs in accordance with the tension view is to register what people actually strive for. To assess human needs in accordance with the teleological view is to assess what things are necessary in order to realize a certain goal (the goal could be, for instance, living a decent life). Assessing what people need (the object of need) in accordance with these views may therefore give totally different results.[1]

The way of looking upon need as a tension in the organism has been questioned. Some people think it is an inadequate use of the term 'need' (Thomson, 1987). Furthermore, it seems to be difficult to avoid completely a teleological view of need.

Abraham Maslow, famous for his hierarchy of needs (Maslow, 1970), can serve as an example here. Some of Maslow's expressions can be interpreted in such a way that he believes that the food, security, belongingness, etc. are needed in order to maintain *health*. Thus Maslow expresses a teleological view where health is the goal of need.[2] What is most troublesome, however, about the tension need is its limited scope. The class of things that people may have a tension need for is quite restricted. It is easy, for instance, to think of a tension need for food and water, but difficult to think of such a need for health care or social benefit. The teleological view of need may therefore be considered as more reasonable as a foundation for analysing the concept of health care need, and any other societal need for that matter.

There is, however, also a third way of using the term 'need', which must not pass without comment. It is possible to say that a wheelchair is a need of Mr Smith's, or that food or love is a human need. The term need here refers to the object needed (X in the formula above). It is important not to forget the distinction between a need (either a tension or a gap) and the object of need (something necessary for eliminating the tension or the gap). There seem to be no restrictions on what things people can need (except impossible things), and any overlooking of the distinction between the need and the object of need might lead to confusion and to the view that need is something very complex and simply indefinable. (This is outlined in Moum (1994).)

The teleological need

The adherents of the teleological tradition, who consider need as a gap, specify the concept somewhat differently. But they all take the view that need is something goal-related – X is needed when X is necessary in

---

[1] The two views of need are discussed in Springborg (1981).

[2] The following quotation illustrates Maslow's teleological view of needs, where the goal is some kind of state of health: Basic needs are human goods that 'are not only wanted and desired by all human beings, but also needed in the sense that they are necessary to avoid illness and psychopathology' (Maslow, 1970, p. xiii).

order to realize a *goal* (Wiggins, 1987). This may be expressed formally in the following way:

P has a need for X in situation S if, and only if, (i) there is a difference in S between the actual state of P and a goal G, and (ii) X is in S a necessary condition (means) for attaining G.

According to this definition there is a need when condition (i) is fulfilled, and a need for X when (i) and (ii) are fulfilled. The term need here refers to the difference – a gap or a state of deficiency.

The goal component plays an important role in the concept. First, the goal *determines* the object of need (that is, the thing needed). The goal 'to live as a farmer' generates a set of needs which partly differs from the set generated by the goal 'to live as a lawyer in the city'. Different goals generate different sets of needs. A clearly defined goal is therefore a prerequisite for a reasonable assessment of needs.

Second, the goal is the *justifying* component in the need concept (Barry, 1965). Claims of need have a special force in most cultures. Perhaps 'P has a need for X' exercises a greater force than 'P wants X'. And if it does, it is not because X in itself is considered valuable, but because X is necessary in order to reach a goal – which is considered valuable. (And in a longer need-chain containing subgoals it is the final goal which is considered intrinsically valuable.) Claims of need get their force from the desirability or value of the goal. This explains why it is normally considered as more important to meet the need for food (in order to survive) than the need for an ice cream (in order to get refreshment).[3]

When the goal is a moral value, the goal of need becomes a source of moral obligation. It may then be argued that there is a *prima facie* obligation to satisfy the basic needs of people, or that people have a *prima facie* right to satisfy their basic needs (Wartofsky, 1992). The basic assumption behind these arguments is that the moral obligation is generated not by the object of need (the thing needed) but by the goal of need.

The teleological view of the general concept of need may be summarized in the following formula: there is a need when the goal is not realized and there is a need of a certain thing when this is necessary

---

[3] There is no agreement on what constitutes the goal of a human need. Different proposals are presented in Liss (1994).

for realizing the goal. This formula may be used in characterizing not only a need for health care but also every other kind of need: a particular thing is needed in so far as it is necessary for eliminating a certain gap or realizing a certain goal.

A health care need is a particular kind of need. According to the basic formula of need, health care is needed in so far as this is necessary for realizing a certain goal. The crucial question is which goal would be realized by satisfying a health care need. This goal cannot be discovered. The goal has to be chosen: a decision has to be made, but the decision need not be arbitrary. It may be based on a rational approach related to the purpose of the health care system. For instance, if good health is the goal of the health care system and if the system should be determined only by the needs of the population, it would be quite irrational not to choose health as the goal of health care need. Therefore, the following preliminary view of health care need may be agreed on: health care is needed in so far as it is necessary for realizing health.[4]

However, this view of health care need is too incomplete to be useful as a foundation for a model for assessing the need. A decision must be made concerning the degree of health that should constitute the goal of health care need. The concept of health must now be analysed. There are different views as to how health should be looked upon. As a consequence it is not sufficient to choose health as a goal. A particular *concept of health* must be chosen. There are mainly two different kinds of perspectives on health: an analytical and a holistic perspective.

The concept of health

In the *analytical perspective of health*, statistical normality is the key concept. Humans have certain characteristics concerning both structure and function. It can be observed how these characteristics contribute to the survival of the individual or to the survival of the species. A species-typical design appears. Scientists can detect the species-typical design of humans by inspecting a large sample of human beings, by making a biostatistical analysis. For instance, the species-typical pulse rate of

---

[4] The goal of medicine is discussed in Nordenfelt and Tengland (1996).

humans consists of that range within which most human heartbeats can be found.[5]

A main thought in the analytical perspective is that there is a disease if the function of an organ deviates in a subnormal way from the species-typical function. The whole person is ill if he or she has an organ which functions subnormally. Health is then defined in terms of disease: a person is in good health if he or she has no disease (Boorse, 1977).

The *holistic perspective on health* takes an opposite starting point. The function and activity of the entire person is conclusive for the judgement of a person's health. Particulars are important only as causal factors behind the functioning of the whole. An everyday formulation of this holistic idea is that a person is healthy if he or she feels well and can function in his or her social context. Here health is the more basic concept, and disease is defined in terms of health. Diseases are characterized as those bodily and mental states or processes that tend to compromise health.

The advantages and disadvantages of these two views of health have been assessed elsewhere. A detailed analysis has demonstrated that the biostatistical theory has serious defects and that it cannot adequately reflect the concept of health either in ordinary discourse or in medical practice (Nordenfelt, 1987). This is a reason for making a choice in favour of the holistic type of analysis.[6]

A holistic theory of health

The basic idea in the holistic theory is simple. Health is defined as a person's ability to reach his or her vital goals (Nordenfelt, 1987). If there is some vital goal the person cannot reach, then he or she lacks health to some degree. In this theory, ability is not something which is characterized statistically. The ability is related to the vital goals of the individual.

The vital goals are related to happiness. The general idea is that the vital goals of humans are the attainment of those states of affairs necessary for happiness. Happiness must here be understood in a general sense, covering such notions as satisfaction, contentedness and pleasure. The holistic concept of health can be characterized in the following way.

[5] The two views are presented in Nordenfelt (1993).
[6] An account of health care need built on the analytical concept of health is presented in Daniels (1985).

P is in good health if, and only if, P is able, given standard circumstances in his or her environment, to fulfil those goals which are necessary and jointly sufficient for his or her minimal happiness (Nordenfelt, 1987).

This holistic concept of health involves a certain relation between health and happiness. It is worth noticing this relation. Health is not happiness, it is only a condition for happiness. But it is not a necessary condition. A person need not be in good health in order to be happy. The person may have his or her vital goals realized by the contribution of others. Neither is health sufficient for happiness. Health defined as a holistic concept is a range of abilities to do certain things. A person may have all the abilities required for him or her to do what is important, but nevertheless not be happy because he or she has not used the ability.

The holistic concept of health is not an either/or concept: it is a dimensional concept. This means that there are different degrees of health: a person may be either more or less healthy. The concept is defined as ability to realize vital goals. The extent to which a person has this ability may vary from time to time, and the degree of health may differ between persons because they differ with respect to their ability to realize their vital goals. This means that the definition of health care need must be further specified concerning the degree of health that should constitute the goal of health care need. It is not reasonable to expect that complete health should be possible in every instance. Optimal health may therefore constitute the goal of health care need.

The concept of health care need

The goal of need is a significant component of the concept of need. Optimal health is a reasonable goal of health care need, and the concept of health care need may be defined in the following way:

P has a need for health care in situation S if, and only if, (a) there is in S a difference between the actual state of P and P's optimal state of health, and (b) health care is necessary in S in order to realize P's optimal state of health.

The actual state here refers to a certain state of health, either of the individual or of the population (if P designates a population). This is the state that is normally checked in a medical examination or in a health control, or by epidemiological measures. Condition (a) in the definition implies that when a person is in a state of health which in a negative way differs from the goal state, he or she has a need. This need may be called a health-related need. In other words, a person has a health-related need in so far as his or her actual state of health is considered unsatisfactory with regard to the optimal state of health. Condition (b) specifies the object of need – that is, what is needed. It implies that there is a need of *health care* in so far as health care is necessary in order to realize the optimal state of health.

The division of the concept of health care need into two components (specified by (a) and (b)) will have some interesting implications both for the setting of priorities in accordance with need, and for the assessment of need. The setting of priorities requires the ranking of needs, and this means the ranking of the health-related need. In order to assess whether there is a need for *health care*, the health-related need must first be assessed.

Three ways of ranking health care needs

It is impossible to meet every need when allocating scarce resources in accordance with need. It might then be found necessary to assign priority to certain categories of needs. Assigning priority in accordance with need means that the needs should be met in a certain order: a more urgent need should be met before a less urgent need. While it is easy to reach agreement on this, it is more difficult to reach agreement on the most urgent need. But a ranking of needs becomes necessary if priority should be assigned in accordance with need in a situation of scarcity. The question is in what way that this should be done.

Need is a difference between an actual state and a goal. The character of this difference varies between one health care need and another. The ranking of health care needs means in principle a ranking of this difference – that is, a ranking of the health-related need. There are several ways of doing this, which implies, of course, that the principle 'in accordance with need' may be used in various senses. This may be illustrated by the following three interpretations.

There is a health-related need, according to the view of health care need just presented, when there is a difference or a gap between the actual state of health and the optimal state of health. There is a need for health care if health care is necessary for eliminating the gap. As the actual state and the optimal state vary between persons and circumstances, the need may be ranked in accordance with the size of the gap. The greater the size, the greater the need. Compare two persons, A and B. Both have a need for health care, but, given scarce resources, only one need can be met. Their actual states are similar, that is, they are ill to the same degree, but their optimal health differs. A can reach a higher state of health than can B. The gap is greater in A's case, which means that A has a greater need for health care than B. Now, if priorities are to be set in accordance with the size of the need, then A should be treated.

A second way of ranking needs would be to consider the consequences of not meeting the needs. The worse the consequences, the more urgent the needs. Compare two persons A and B, whose needs cannot both be met. Both are ill to the same degree, but the consequences of not meeting the needs differ. Not meeting the need of A means that A's condition deteriorates substantially, and A ends up in a low state of health. Not meeting the need of B means hardly any change in B's condition. A's need is more urgent than B's need. Treating A and not treating B in this case means that the health care is allocated in accordance with the more urgent need.

A third way of ranking health care needs would be to focus mainly on the actual states of health, and give priority to the needs which derive from the lowest states of health. The intuitively reasonable idea here is that scarce health care resources should first be allocated to those who are most ill; that the more ill they are the more important are the needs. Suppose, for example, that both A and B are ill, but A is much more ill than B, that is, the actual state of health of A is much lower than the actual state of health of B. In this case A has a more important need than B, and if the health care should be allocated in accordance with the importance of the need, A should be treated.

These three ways of ranking needs are not the only methods; there are others (Liss, 1993). This means that a choice has to be made as to which ranking is to be used when assigning priority in accordance with health care need. This choice may be based on a certain principle or criterion in order to avoid arbitrariness. It might be a matter of debate by what principle the principle of need should then be accompanied, but it is hardly debatable that it must be thus accompanied. The conclusion to be drawn is that the principle of need cannot alone constitute a criterion for the allocation of scarce health care resources. The setting of priorities *exclusively* in accordance with need in a situation of scarcity is not possible.

A model for assessing health care needs

The concept of health care need has three fundamental components: the actual state, the goal of health care need, and the object of health care need. Information about these components is necessary and sufficient for an assessment of health care need. The leading idea in the model is then to obtain this information. The procuration may be performed in three stages.

1 Determine the actual state.
2 Determine the goal of health care need.
3 Determine the object of need.

The order of the first two steps might be reversed. The third step, however, cannot be carried out before the first and second are finished. An assessment of health care need, in accordance with this design, may be carried out both at the micro and the macro level. It is possible to assess both an individual and a population need for health care by carrying out the three stages.

The *actual state* refers to the person's actual ability to realize his or her vital goals. To determine the actual state at the first stage means to determine the person's ability in this respect. A kind of survey approach may be used for this purpose. Mainly, two different types are conceivable – interviews or questionnaires, and clinical examinations. Perhaps the use of interviews or questionnaires is an inexpensive method, but the clinical examination seems to be the most informative method. Based on a clearly defined concept of health care need, and properly used, it may yield all the information sufficient for an assessment, including the ranking, of health care needs.

A certain state of health constitutes the *goal of health care need*. It is not possible to reach full health in every instance. A decision therefore has to be made concerning what degree of health should constitute the goal of health care need, that is, the optimal state of health. That a certain state of health constitutes the goal of need means that when this state is realized, the need is satisfied and no further action is required. A need is basically a difference or a gap between the actual state and a goal. Satisfying a need therefore means the elimination of this difference or gap. The need is eliminated when the difference or gap is eliminated. There is, however, more than one way or eliminating a need. The gap can be eliminated either by manipulating the actual state or by changing the goal, or both. The first thought is to manipulate the actual state, that is, to give care or cure, but it is in principle possible to eliminate a need by choosing a very low state of health. The goal could be lowered from, for instance, 'fit for work' to 'manage all right at home'.

It is possible then, but hardly acceptable, to cut down dramatically the scope of a population's need of health care by using a certain concept of need, (a concept which mirrors low ambitions with respect to the goal). It is also possible to do the opposite. High ambitions could be used with respect to the goal, which would mean an increased amount of health care need among the population. If the ambitions are related to medical progress, a population's need of care remains constant even if more diseases are cured.[7]

How should the right degree of health now be determined? There is no algorithm for this. The goal has to be chosen, and the choice is not only a matter of empirical investigation but also, and mainly, a matter of evaluation. The choice may be dependent upon some basic evaluation on the part of the chooser. This implies that there is an issue at the second stage that may be considered as a key-issue for the whole assessment procedure. Who shall have a dominating influence on the decisions: whose values should determine the choice of the goal, that is, the optimal state of health? Two perspectives dominate the discourse on need assessments – the client's and the provider's (Hunt, McEwen and McKenna, 1985). The client's or individual's own specification of the goal might be obtained by interviews or questionnaires, probably in very general terms. An alternative is to let the individual directly identify the health-related need (the difference or gap). The specified goal may be implicitly expressed in such cases. The provider's specification may be obtained in almost the same ways. Perhaps a

---

[7] The social insurance system in many countries contains an easily manipulable goal. Within such a system a subsistence level is specified in monetary terms. The subsistence level, which is a politically chosen level and therefore in a sense easily manipulable, constitutes the goal of need (for social benefit). A person whose means fall below this level is considered to have a need and is entitled to help from the system.

specified goal is implicitly expressed when health care need is assessed in ordinary clinical examinations.

There is, in addition, at least a third party – the ordinary citizen. There are different methods by which the values of the citizen may be considered, but perhaps these values are best considered in a well-ordered representative democracy. The powers of the citizen may be delegated to health authorities. However, medical and other types of professional knowledge are necessary in order to ensure that the specified goal will be realistic. Perhaps the issue of a specified goal of health care need should be settled in a joint venture between, for instance, lay persons, politicians, health personnel and administrators.

The determination of the *object of health care need* at the third stage concerns the services needed (the necessary treatment or resources for realizing the goal). The determination at this stage is to a great extent, but not completely, an issue for different professionals. The situation varies with the number of treatments available for a specific purpose. There may, of course, be only one treatment available, or none at all, but in many cases there is a choice, including the possibility of renouncing treatment altogether. In making a choice here professional considerations are not the only valid themes. Other values, in particular ethical themes, must play an important part. This speaks in favour of, for instance, the influence of lay persons on the decisions at this stage.

Another interesting issue concerns what factors should be allowed to influence the decision about the goal. Economic considerations constitute one of the most interesting factors here (medical knowledge is another). It is tempting to say that this factor actually should influence the decision. For instance, if only a certain degree of health can be afforded it may seem pointless to choose a higher degree as the goal of health care needed,[8] but to adopt this attitude would be to make a mistake. It is important to distinguish between (i) there is a need, and (ii) this need can or should be met. It is a mistake to argue that there is a need only if it can or should be satisfied: the second condition (ii) should not be put as a necessary condition for the first (i). There is no contradiction in saying that 'There is a need (for X) but this need cannot be satisfied'. Of course a thirsty person in the desert needs water even if there is no water within reach; a starving person needs food even if he or she cannot afford it.

[8] For an argument in this direction see Acheson (1978).

Thus the existence of a health-related need is altogether independent of whether to meet the need can be afforded or not. Economic considerations should not therefore influence the *identification* of needs. They may only influence the decision whether the need should be satisfied or not.

Assessing the population's need for health care

A population's need for health care is equivalent to the sum of the individuals' needs. Mainly there are two ways of adding up the individuals' needs for health care in accordance with the sketched model.

First, it is possible to add up the results from completed assessments at the micro level. The three stages are carried out for each individual and the assessments can be added up in terms of different categories of health care needs. An assessment of the individual's need is in a sense a decentralized assessment, but it is also possible to assess health care need at a more centralized level. The need for health care may finally be assessed by, for instance, a health authority, a committee or a health council. The suggested model may then be used at the macro level. The adding up in this case does not concern the result of a completed assessment but the foundation for a centralized assessment. Every stage is added up separately. In practice this means adding up the results from the determination of the actual states, expressed, for instance, in terms of different categories or states of ill health. The remaining two stages may likewise be described in corresponding categories. The result of a completed assessment may then be expressed in terms of different categories of health care need.

Various methods may be used to obtain information about the actual state – the health status of the population. A certain kind of survey approach might be suggested; for instance, a representative sample of the population could be examined regarding their health status.

The goal of health care need varies with different diseases or states of ill health – the optimal state of health is instantiated by different degrees of health. The goal must then be specified for every different category of state of ill health. The actors may be the same as were involved at the micro level.

This sketch is a first step towards a complete model for an assessment of health care need. In its present state it leaves many questions unanswered, particularly about matters of measurement. However, the sketch is sufficiently substantial for the advantages to become evident. The assessment is divided into three stages. This has two significant implications. First, the distinction between the need and the object of need is upheld. It is then possible, for instance, to identify a health-related need (the difference between the actual state and the goal) without any influence from knowledge about necessary treatment (its cost, its effectiveness, etc.).

Second, the goal of need is given attention at a separate stage. This means that the main value-laden component in the concept of health care need is made public. In the sketched model the settlement of the value-laden issue at stage two is a prerequisite of an adequate assessment of health care need.

References

Acheson, R. M. (1978) The definition and identification of need for health care. *Journal of Epidemiology and Community Health*, **32**, 10–15.

Barry, B. (1965) *Political Argument*. London: Routledge & Kegan Paul.

Boorse, C. (1977) Health as a theoretical concept. *Philosophy of Science*, **44**, 542–573.

Daniels, N. (1985) *Just Health Care*. Cambridge: Cambridge University Press.

Hunt, S., McEwen, J., McKenna, S. (1985) Measuring health status: a new tool for clinicians and epidemiologists. *Journal of the Royal College of General Practitioners*, **35**, 185–188.

Liss, P-E. (1993) *Health Care Need*. Aldershot: Avebury.

Liss, P-E. (1994) On need and quality of life. In *Concepts and Measurement of Quality of Life in Health Care* (L. Nordenfelt, ed.). Dordrecht: Kluwer Academic Publishers.

Maslow, A. H. (1970) *Motivation and Personality*, 2nd edn. New York: Harper & Row.

Moum, T. (1994) Needs, rights and resources in quality of life research. In *Concepts and Measurement of Quality of Life in Health Care* (L. Nordenfelt, ed.). Dordrecht: Kluwer Academic Publishers.

Nordenfelt, L. (1987) *On the Nature of Health*. Dordrecht: D. Reidel Publishing Company.

Nordenfelt, L. (1993) *Quality of Life, Health and Happiness*. Aldershot: Avebury.

Nordenfelt, L., Tengland, P-A. (eds) (1996) *The Goals and Limits of Medicine*. Stockholm: Almqvist & Wiksell International.

Springborg, P. (1981) *The Problems of Human Needs and the Critique of Civilisation*. London: George Allen & Unwin.

Thomson, G. (1987) *Needs*. London: Routledge & Kegan Paul.

Wartotsky, M. (1992) The social presuppositions of medical knowledge. In *The Ethics of Diagnosis* (J. L. Peset and D. Gracia, eds). Dordrecht: Kluwer Academic Publishers.

Wiggins, D. (1987) *Needs, Values, Truth*. Oxford: Basil Blackwell.

Chapter 3
Assessment of need and case management: an evolving concept

Peter A. Woods and Steve Baldwin

Introduction

Case management as a concept began life in the USA as a means of addressing the difficulties posed by the existence of fragmented services and partial funding by insurance companies (Sevick, 1990). Its essential components involved the pooling of resources, linking their provision to assessed need, and adoption of a holistic approach with clearly defined objectives. Intagliata (1982) described the elements of case management as including: (a) comprehensive assessment of individual needs; (b) developing an individual plan of care to meet those identified needs; (c) procuring an individualized 'package' of care services; (d) monitoring and evaluating the quality of services and outcomes; and (e) offering long-term, flexible support, information and counselling.

In the UK, Pilling (1988) offered the definition:

> Essentially a case manager is an expert who connects a client with all the relevant services. To perform the connecting service efficiently the case manager fully assesses the client's needs, discusses with the client a plan of action and, if necessary, performs an advocacy function. The final stage is one of monitoring to make sure the services are properly implemented (p. 7).

Nonetheless, despite widespread popularity among several professional groups, including social work, nursing and clinical psychology, some reservations have recently been expressed about the limits of case management implementation (e.g. Onyett, 1992). Some critics have suggested that 'case management' lacks definitional precision. Moreover, its exponents may not have adequately explored the underlying value systems and assumptions on which it is founded.

Needs assessment has been offered as one opportunity to specify more exactly the interface between behavioural methods and service implementation. The central axis of needs assessment in practice is the attempt to provide services to meet human needs, rather than resolve problems. Although the debate about the definition of 'needs' has been similarly sterile, the concept has been accepted by a wide range of professionals (Baldwin, 1987). Thus, clinical psychologists, social workers, nurses and occupational therapists have introduced needs assessment methods to replace less comprehensive systems in clinical and educational settings.

Unfortunately, however, most needs assessments also lack precision and clarity. Also, there has been little consensus about what passes for a 'needs assessment'. Even within the same service system, professionals may adopt different methodologies, and yet use similar terms to describe their efforts.

The concepts of case management and needs assessment therefore merit closer inspection, to determine their utility as the means by which to organize human services in the 1990s and beyond.

The social policy context

In the UK, the White Paper *Caring for People* (Department of Health, 1989) had been considerably influenced by the Griffiths Report (1988) and the Audit Commission (1989) with its emphasis upon resource rationing as an essential component of case management, stating that: 'The government also sees advantages in linking case management with delegated responsibility for budgetary management' (3.3.5). Views in the White Papers about case management included the need to adopt a client-centred approach, with individual needs-based assessment, and they encouraged client involvement in the process of planning and securing the delivery of care. They also encouraged local authority social services departments, through the case management process, to build an individual's package of care from a 'mixed economy' of service providers. In so doing case management is placed firmly in a free enterprise market culture with a primary concern for cost-effectiveness.

Both the White Paper and subsequent legislation (NHS and Community Care Act, 1990) stressed the need for structural changes in which the local authority as a 'service purchaser' would become less involved in 'service provision', the latter being increasingly supplied by the voluntary and private sector. As part of this dichotomy of function, emphasis has been placed upon the need for case managers to adopt a predominantly procurement role with little or no involvement in direct service provision. The latter function has been a source of much tension in several case management systems.

What is case management?

An examination of recent reviews of case management implementation confirms that no single accepted definition exists. In the USA, the term has been used to describe several related functions performed by a case manager, including: information provision; referral; review; access to services; advocacy; counselling; monitoring. This wide remit has been extended in some services to include highly specialist activities such as psychotherapy, although this is generally perceived as too much involvement for a generic worker. Most work in this area involves a clear procurement role for case managers, and it is this potential conflict of interest which remains inadequately specified in many human service systems. Although this central dilemma has been acknowledged in some reviews (Renshaw, 1988) it has not been satisfactorily resolved at the level of practice.

Austin and O'Connor (1989), in an extensive literature review, acknowledged that a wide range of practice can be accommodated within the general frame of case management, and suggested a continuum of case management activities along which any one approach could be placed. The two poles of the continuum can be conceptualized as: (a) one where greater emphasis is placed upon financial responsibilities in which the case-managers are budget-holding service purchasers who stand autonomous from provision, function as gatekeepers with an emphasis on cost containment, and the monitoring of service delivery systems, and (b), at the other pole, case managers are not themselves budget holders with the corresponding resource rationing responsibilities, but are independent 'service brokers' (Salisbury, Dickey and Crawford, 1987) who develop a 'working alliance' (Brechin and Swaine, 1988) with their clients (to whom their first loyalty goes) and whose principal functions are to coordinate care planning and service delivery, with an emphasis on advocacy.

Care Management is the term that was adopted in the UK (because 'case' was considered offensive to service users), and the model advocated in the *Caring for People* White Paper was widely introduced. The model could be described as an 'extended brokerage case management' (Holloway *et al.*, 1991), which was seen as affording client protection:

> Care Managers should, in effect, act as brokers for services across the statutory and independent sectors. They should not, therefore, be involved in direct service delivery; nor should they normally carry managerial responsibility for the services they arrange. This removes any possible conflict of interest... (Department of Health, 1989).

Role confusion

The confusion between procurement and enabling roles has long been at the heart of criticisms of case management systems. There are some, such as Dowson (1990), who argue that the conflicts of interest and biases generated by undertaking specific roles are such that they can only be avoided by ensuring that each of the following four functions should be undertaken by separate agencies which should be mutually independent of each other: (a) service funding/purchasing; (b) service brokerage; (c) advocacy; and (d) service provision.

Briggs (1991) has observed that there is an implicit assumption in the White Paper and community care legislation that the coming together of a case manager and client is that of two equals doing business together. However, he points out that it is naive to assume equality in a 'helper–helped' relationship if one party controls resources that the other party needs. Similarly, the notion that case managers can operate as '... neutral, unaligned sources of pertinent information and also as conduits for the flow of information ...' (Müeller and Hopp, 1987) is an untested naive assumption about the value-neutrality of case managers.

Ovretveit (1991) has reviewed several models for case management teams that have evolved in the UK in recent years. He noted one that goes some way towards resolving the 'efficient economic use of resources versus creation of a high quality, individually tailored service' conflict in which the case management team leader is a budget holder who does not delegate it to the case management practitioners. The latter act as case coordinators or service brokers who apply to the team leader to 'buy' certain services for their clients (Richardson and Higgins, 1990). However, the employment relationship between them does not entirely remove the dilemma.

In an interesting review of a case management project in Wakefield, Richardson and Higgins (1990) quoted one case manager who described the job as 'working on ball bearings'. Although the case management team (of social workers) was set up with the assumption that case managers would undertake an 'advocacy' role on behalf of clients, they were under clear pressure to meet certain expectations of their employing authority (the service purchaser). They argued that great resilience is essential to cope with the inevitable ambiguities and uncertainties that arise in an extremely demanding job.

Another area of confusion about role separation involves the extent to which the information-giving and counselling roles of case managers might develop into a relationship with the client which provides therapeutic support and could be construed as the provision of psychotherapy. A strict interpretation of the White Paper concept of case management would argue that there is a potential conflict of interest between a procurement role and a psychotherapist role, and that the two roles cannot or should not be mixed. However, others argue strongly that case managers should consciously cultivate the therapeutic aspects of their relationships with their clients in order to help them engage more readily in the assessment of need and individual care planning processes (e.g. Harris and Bergman, 1987).

This aspect of the debate about the role of case managers is perhaps assisted by reference to the schematic representation of case management work and service provision work shown in Figure 3.1. The two circles are meant to encompass all activities construed as being case management work (e.g. needs assessment, shared action planning, service procurement) and service provision work (e.g. residential support, supported employment, everyday living skill training), respectively. However, the shaded area is where the two broad categories of activity overlap and would include such activities as counselling, assertion and self-esteem encouragement, and aspects of psychotherapy.

There can be no single, universally accepted definition of case management. Ideally each project should state quite clearly where its boundaries lie. Shepherd (1990) has pointed out that '...in most situations, both 'managerial' [pure] and 'clinical' [overlap with service provision] elements of case management will be present simultaneously. Funding agencies, however, must be clear as to exactly what kind of case management service they expect, as this has both training and resource implications' (p. 60). To this it might be added that it also has

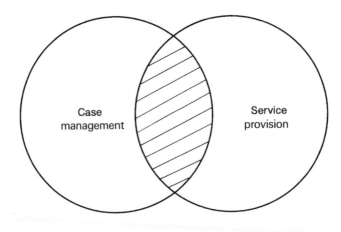

Figure 3.1 Case management and service provision activities

recruitment implications, with many social workers and psychologists (and other care professionals) not wishing to drop totally the core therapeutic skills they have to offer.

In many mental health services the 'brokerage case management' model was said to have limited value in relation to care of people with chronic mental health problems. A response to this has been the growth of 'clinical case management' (Franklin *et al.*, 1994), especially in the USA, which stresses the importance of small case-loads and a broad clinical remit. In the UK the term 'clinical case management' is often used interchangeably with 'assertive community treatment' (Burns and Santos, 1995) and is characterized by individualized treatments, programmatic flexibility, care of the most severely mentally ill, inter-agency cooperation and continuity of care (Burns, 1997).

Some case management systems have included principles by which to organize service provision. Two common principles include provision at the lowest (i.e. least invasive) level of intervention, and establishment of the least restrictive environment for the client (Müeller and Hopp, 1987). Although consonant with some prevailing service ideologies, these principles frequently have remained buried beneath an administrative bureaucracy. Thus, in practice, the implementation of new frameworks has not always impacted on the deeper structural system problems.

Evaluative research findings

Due to the recent development of case management services, few formal evaluations of effectiveness have been completed. Most published studies have been restricted to descriptive accounts of an individual service in a single location. To date, few comparative evaluations between (or within) services have been documented, and this remains an unexplored research area. The challenge for evaluators is to move from demonstration studies to focus on whole service systems. As yet, however, an adequate methodology for this has not been developed.

One study in the USA investigated the cost-benefits of case management services to a cohort of hospitalized people with mental health problems (Müeller and Hopp, 1987). In this service, social work gerontologists were employed to provide a range of services, including referral, follow-up, advocacy and counselling. Service plans were completed for individuals, following completion of checklists of problems and strengths; 20 clients were monitored for an average of 15 months, with a focus on outcome.

The study produced several themes which have recurred in subsequent investigations. First, the lack of clarity about the status of the case manager in the system produced role ambiguity both for these workers, and for other personnel in the service. For example, in some situations case managers had a responsibility to identify a deficit in the system, and were also required to provide the solution to the problem. Second, short regular counselling sessions from the case manager were sufficient to prevent relapse (and subsequent readmission) among discharged clients. Third, the case management system may have assisted in the prevention of readmission of clients into hospital.

In the UK, a case management service was established for elderly people in the local neighbourhood (Davies and Challis, 1986). Case managers were required to complete needs assessments of clients, and provide direct services where appropriate. These services included counselling, as well as provision of aids, adaptations and access to other services; workers were required to record their inputs precisely, as well as to monitor the impact of their contributions.

Case workers in this service were expected to provide an input to approximately 30 clients; this contrasts with other services, where the variation of caseload size has ranged from three to 250. The extent of involvement from a case worker will depend on the size of caseload; to maintain quality, an upper limit on the number of clients represented by one worker should be established at management level.

The Camden and Islington Case Manager Project, a pilot scheme for people with all types of physical disability, was evaluated by the Rehabilitation Resource Centre at City University (Pilling, 1988) which concluded, from a questionnaire survey of service users, that better services had been obtained as a consequence of case management intervention. The case managers were given a considerable degree of 'independence' which was seen as a strength: '...making it more effective as an advocate and more acceptable as a mediator. Independence also gave it freedom to make contacts without restrictions from hierarchical authorities or professional boundaries' (p. 9).

Richardson and Higgins (1990) reported on their study of the Wakefield Case Management Project noting that '...if it will work here, it will work anywhere' (p. 23). Set up under the assumption that case managers would undertake an advocacy role on behalf of their clients, providing needs-led services rather than a resource-constrained one, they concluded that such services can only be established with some offset costs. Case managers found their job both very rewarding, but also very stressful because of the often opposing pressures to meet simultaneously certain expectations of their employing authority and the raised expectations of clients.

The Wakefield Project involved a case management team with an internal structure which split the jobs of client advocacy and budgetary control; the latter was the responsibility of the project coordinator and the former the prime responsibility of the social worker case managers. In their conclusions, Richardson and Higgins (1990) raised a critical issue for consideration in any evaluation of case management:

> It is crucial to distinguish the process – what case managers do – from the content – what they achieve... It is possible to imagine a good case management service which achieves little in effect, because resources are particularly constrained... Conversely, it is [also] possible to imagine a bad case management service which achieves a lot, simply because the relevant authorities were awash with spare resources which happened to be put in clients' directions (p. 25).

Clinical case management and particularly the 'Programme for Assertive Community Treatment' (PACT), has been described in detail and subjected to over thirteen randomized controlled trials (Burns and

Santos, 1995). These found the PACT approach reduced the need for in-patient care and increased 'community tenure'; the latter was loosely equated with avoidance of relapse. Furthermore, costs of the experimental service were found to be partially or totally met by the in-patient reductions of inpatient costs (Dincin *et al.*, 1993).

Skills

The five main components of case management described by Intagliata (1982) have associated core skills: (a) assessment; (b) individual service planning; (c) administrative/financial aspects of procurement; (d) counselling and psychotherapy and (e) monitoring and evaluation. Although there has been some debate about the way in which these separate functions are integrated by the same person (Fisher, Landis and Clark, 1988), these core activities define the role of the case manager in service systems.

Assessment

The process of case management is contingent on an initial set of statements about the perceived needs of clients. There has been considerable debate about the ability of clients to define and assert their own needs. Typically, this function has been viewed as one of the central activities of the case manager. Hence, despite the recognition that the user of services should ideally specify the service responses, in practice this task has been completed by staff. Some of the new budgetary arrangements, however, will move some clients closer to this ideal.

Unfortunately, no procedures have achieved widespread currency in human services, and this process of needs assessment has remained idiosyncratic and ill-defined. In many services, it has been restricted to the reduplication of existing service options. 'Assessment' has been limited to the provision of already-available options, rather than the identification of new services. Arguably, the process of assessment should also identify service options for the user not already in existence.

Individual service planning

For those client groups who have a range of additional special needs (especially those with intellectual disability), coordination of individual service planning is a major component function for case managers. At the 'service management' pole, this function tends to focus on an Individual program planning (IPP) meeting attended by various contributors to the assessment of need process that the case manager chairs (e.g. Jenkins, Felce, Toogood, Mansell and de Kock, 1988). At the 'client advocacy' pole, less emphasis is placed on large meetings with greater attention given to the development of a relationship between the client and case manager in this process e.g. Open University's shared action planning (Brechin and Swaine, 1986, 1987) which has been described as:

> A radical approach to shared assessment, which emphasises the importance of getting to know and understand each other; the identification of aims in terms of what people would like to see happening; and a process of considering plans for action which recognises the existence of different perspectives, moves the focus away from the usual concern with the individual and how he/she should change, to focus instead on the role of other people and wider circumstances (p. 224) (Brechin and Swaine, 1988).

Administrative/financial aspects of procurement

This may be *the* core function of case management activity. More than the other skilled activities, the provision of administrative and financial techniques is central to the service procurement function. Moreover, the job descriptions of some case managers will revolve around these functions, with a focus on allocation of resources within a *fixed* budget.

Counselling and psychotherapy

Many accounts of implementation attempts have included the counselling of clients as a core activity for case managers (Fisher, Landis and Clark, 1988; Müeller and Hopp, 1987). This activity is based on regular interaction with the client, for problem-solving sessions, or to resolve unmet psychological needs. Often, such contact develops into a preventive role, to assist clients to remain in local neighbourhoods following discharge (Davies and Challis, 1986).

Despite the commonplace development of counselling roles for case managers, it remains unclear whether this activity is compatible with the other defined functions. Without clear boundaries, 'counselling' can easily become 'psychotherapy', not least when vulnerable and at-risk client populations are involved. Also, there may be an inherent role conflict between the nature of counselling and the functions of administration/finance. A client may become depressed about the lack of services to meet their needs; they may find it difficult to discuss this in a counselling session, with the same staff member who is responsible for that provision.

Although several case management programmes have included psychotherapy functions with clients, many problems have developed in this context. First, many case managers have no background or training in psychotherapy, and may have exceeded their professional competence. Second, the role conflict between service provider and psychotherapist is potentially damaging for both staff and clients. Third, staff appointed to case manager posts may not wish to offer such services to their clients. Fourth, psychotherapy provision by case managers may not be cost-effective or desirable.

Monitoring and evaluation

Another major function that case managers are well-placed to under-take (and the more they divest themselves of service provision roles the better) is quality monitoring and evaluation at the individual client level. Through needs assessment and shared action planning they can assist clients to set outcome objectives and determine the process objectives for service providers. As part of their ongoing case management work they can then monitor the performance quality of service providers and evaluate whether quality of life outcome objectives are achieved.

In addition to the debate about the core functions of case manage-ment, there is a second unresolved debate about whether such services should be provided by one person, or several. Hence, in some services, the functions listed above have been provided by one case manager. In other services, these functions have been shared within a team of specialists (Ovretveit, 1991).

This second debate has introduced familiar material about the ability of qualified professionals to manage each other, despite very different backgrounds and training. As yet, there are no definite answers to these questions; other data are required to inform this debate. Reports of services based on a case management approach have yet to include comparisons between the effectiveness of individuals and teams.

Process of needs assessment

Previous reviews of needs assessment have concluded that the lack of precision in definition has precluded advancement in this field. With a lack of consensus even on the meaning of 'need' (Baldwin, 1986, 1998) there has been much debate about how this might relate to 'needs assessment'.

The main area of debate has been about the ability of users to define their own needs. Radical critiques of social policy have suggested that the conflict of interest from professional involvement may prevent any objective assessment of client needs (Illich, 1977). Nonetheless, professionals have continued to assume this role by default in many human services, with only limited assistance or impact from advocacy services. Only the adequate separation of roles of assessor, purchaser and provider will resolve this debate.

Previous attempts at needs assessment often have been limited in potency by inadequate breadth or depth of measurement. Due to restrictions of design, needs assessments previously have been focused on checklists or scorecards. Thus, in some settings, the current activities of clients have been measured against predetermined lists. This approach can be helpful in helping to ensure that an adequate range of activities is considered for assessment. It cannot, however, substitute for more open-ended techniques.

Moreover, although all clients share universal human needs by virtue of their existence (Baldwin, 1986), most clients will have (additional) special needs. The latter will often result from specific aspects of their disabilities, and could also be related to religious, ethnic and other cultural factors (Nadirshaw, 1991). Thus service provision for most users will reflect a mix of generic and special needs (Brewin et al., 1987). To specify this mix adequately, more sophisticated methods of recording than checklists are required.

Not all existing needs assessments have been designed to reflect this complex template of needs. Some methods have been limited by a too narrow focus (Brewin et al., 1987); others have failed to address the theme of needs, and have retained a preoccupation with problem-based assessment.

Other attempts to invoke needs assessment have been restricted by a cookbook approach to measurement of clients. Such strategies are doomed to failure, and risk the integrity of both staff and users. For many staff, needs assessment is merely the most recent of a series of attempts to specify the activities of clients; without adequate training for implementation, needs assessment techniques will also join the already high pile of discarded 'good ideas'.

Although no single method of needs assessment exists, some current methods clearly are inappropriate to the task of determining the template of client requirements. To overcome resistance amongst staff, simple, effective methods will be most likely to succeed. Optimally, recording should be restricted to a single sheet in any one need area (Baldwin, Baser and Harding, 1990; Harding, Baldwin and Baser, 1987).

Interprofessional themes

In the context of new services for a range of client groups in the 1990s, many questions remain unanswered about the relationships between different professional groups. Thus, despite a clear delineation of different health and social services professional groups in the 1980s, the shift from functional to general management imposed a new set of values onto service systems.

Any lack of a clear service structure will produce specific problems for the implementation of case management in the 1990s. The origins of case management in social work services may generate particular problems for health service staff, unused to different lines of accountability. Also, the 'ownership' of case management by specific professional groups may spark further interprofessional rivalries. Shepherd (1990) has noted that:

> The question of which profession is best placed to function as case manager is complicated since the role combines elements of many different mental health professions – social work, nursing, psychiatry, clinical psychology, and occupational therapy. There have even been suggestions of inventing a new profession, but this does not seem practical... Because of the overlap between professional roles, whoever takes on the role of case manager might meet considerable resistance from colleagues: if case managers are to function effectively these issues will have to be addressed (p. 60).

It is inservice training, however, which may hold the key to the future of case management in human services. Specifically, the paucity of formal methods to acquire the prerequisite skills of case management may jeopardize its implementation. At present, much of this implementation is completed by health and social service professionals not specifically trained in this area. One result is that staff are left to impose their own interpretations of the system, without adequate feedback or monitoring. Unfortunately, some systems described as based on 'case management' have become corrupted by loose implementation.

Appropriate implementation of case management would require adoption of agreed local or national guidelines which would reflect specific standards. Ideally these standards would reflect consensus about the skills and experiences required of staff employed as case managers, irrespective of their professional background or origins. Such case management training curricula would reflect a focus on core skills, as well as an inclusion of local factors. Thus, local services would require their staff to demonstrate competence in aspects of case management specific to that service, as well as a range of more general skills.

A very useful first step towards filling this void has been provided by CCETSW's publication, *Assessment, Care Management and Inspection in Community Care; Towards a Practice Curriculum* (Briggs and Weinstein, 1991). As a contribution towards the 'Improving Social Work Education and Training' series, it undertakes a skills analysis of the three functions, examining the training implications and setting out the knowledge and competencies required for various tasks.

Limits to case management

The recent development of the case management concept will exert limitations on its implementation in human services. Already, boundary problems have been identified about the extent to which case management can be distinguished from service provision; some services have deliberately blurred these distinctions (Müeller and Hopp, 1987). Nonetheless, without such distinctions between case management (i.e. need identification) and service provision (i.e. response to this need) staff may fail to complete either role adequately. The role conflict of these functions may make the two jobs incompatible.

Other services have resolved these conflicts with a different response. In the UK, many services have continued to function without recourse to case management methods. Other services have rejected these methods after a brief trial period (Baldwin, 1998). Selection of optimum methods in any single location should be an empirical decision, based on equitable distribution of resources, according to client needs. Case management has been the subject of criticism on the grounds that it meets administrative, rather than clinical, requirements. It may be helpful to managers; clients and staff may be less enthusiastic.

Moreover, case management may be viewed as a return to individualism within service structures. Following the reform of social work services to incorporate wider community and neighbourhood perspectives in the 1980s (Cooper, 1989), this shift to the individual consumer may risk invocation of outdated pathology models. Future successful implementation of case management should address this planning dilemma.

Service brokerage may assist with this dilemma. The separation of consumers from suppliers of human services, essential to avoid conflicts of interest in planning and provision, can be assisted via brokerage systems. Successful establishment of independent mediating structures between consumers and suppliers will be required to overcome chronic problems of 'implementation paradox' (the tendency for staff to meet system, not client, needs).

The mixed economy of provision in the 1990s will require more sophisticated approaches to service planning and design. Any shift to more privatized care will generate a renewed focus on the ability of statutory service managers adequately to establish the primacy of the consumer in the complex template of provision. It remains to be adequately demonstrated that case management can achieve this difficult aim.

Evaluation attempts

The relative recency of case management implementation so far has precluded full evaluation of outcomes. Nonetheless, some early reports of descriptive studies have been completed and not all have been favourable. Marshall *et al.* (1995), for example, found that 'case management' (i.e. brokerage case management) is a costly approach with no obvious benefits for patients. Furthermore, in an editorial in the *Lancet*, Marshall (1995) dubbed case management 'a dubious practice ... underevaluated and ineffective, but new government policy'.

Given the primacy of monitoring and evaluation in the future template of services, the location of case management in the non-government sector seems a very promising development. Unfortunately, however, despite the enthusiasm for case management methods, there have been few signs of investment by managers in evaluation studies. Any shift to locate services in a new structure of case management should be contingent on the prior establishment of a database.

Such databases would include the examination of individual outcomes, as well as a focus on the whole system. To achieve this, more inter-agency collaboration will be required, to ensure access to information from different services and their staff.

Conclusion

Case management is certainly attracting much debate and excitement, but there are definite issues concerning role specification, relationships to service providers and training that need further clarification at both national and local levels. It offers the opportunity to develop greater client involvement and needs-led service planning and generally to 'loosen up' rigid service systems. However, it is only part of the picture which must also include a major commitment by service purchasers to replace traditional, institution-based services with more flexible, community-based services. Also, in the enthusiasm to push ahead with innovative case management approaches, the following words of caution from Shepherd (1990) are salutary:

> ...case management represents the latest in a long line of 'magic' solutions to hit community [services]. Like many good ideas it risks being 'oversold' and then rejected as people become disillusioned that it has failed to live up to expectations. Case management is not a panacea: it is a useful idea which addresses a central problem to do with the coordination and monitoring of community services. It is not a substitute for an adequate range of community provisions (p. 59).

For the future, Burns (1997) has recently stated that

> ...Case management and care management in 10 years' time will probably be very different to what they are now. As with many vigorous ideas, the meaning of case management has evolved rapidly as the context in which it operated has changed and understanding of its functioning developed. A willingness to understand this historical development (and tolerate inevitable future changes and ambiguities) is required if sense is to be made of the burgeoning literature in this field.

References

Audit Commission (1989) *Developing Community Care for Adults with a Mental Handicap*. London: HMSO.

Austin, C., O'Connor, K. (1989) Case management: components and program contexts. In M. E. Peterson and D. White (eds) *Health Care of the Elderly*. New York: Sage.

Baldwin, S. (1986) Problems with needs – where theory meets practice. *Disability, Handicap and Society*, 1(2), 139–145.

Baldwin, S. (1987) From community to neighbourhoods. *Disability, Handicap and Society*, 2(1), 41–59.

Baldwin, S. (1998) *Needs Assessment and Community Care*. Oxford: Butterworth-Heinemann.

Baldwin, S., Baser, C., Harding, K. (1990) *Multi-level Needs Assessments*. London: British Association of Behavioural Psychotherapy.

Brechin, A., Swaine, J. (1986) Shared action planning: a skills workbook. In *Mental Handicap: Patterns for Living*. Milton Keynes: Open University Press.

Brechin, A., Swaine, J. (1987) *Changing Relationships: Shared Action Planning with People with a Mental Handicap*. Harper and Row: London.

Brechin, A., Swaine, J. (1988) Professional/client relationships: creating a 'working alliance' with people with learning difficulties. *Disability, Handicap and Society*, 3(3), 213–226.

Brewin, C., Wing, J. K., Mangen, S. P., Brugha, T. S., MacCarthy, B. (1987) Principles and practice of measuring needs in the long-term mentally ill: the MRC needs for care assessment. *Psychological Medicine*, 17, 971–982.

Burns, B. J. (1997) Case management, care management and care programming. *British Journal of Psychiatry*, 170, 393–395.

Burns, B. J., Santos, A. B. (1995). Assertive community treatment; an update of randomized trials. *Psychiatric Services*, 46, 669–675.

Briggs, S. (1991) Community care, case management and the psychodynamic perspective. *Journal of Social Work Practice*, 5(1), 71–81.

Briggs, S., Weinstein, J. (1991) *Assessment, Case Management and Inspection in Community Care*. London: CCETSW.

Cooper, J. (1989) From casework to community care: the end is where we start from. *British Journal of Social Work*, 19, 177–188.

Davies, B., Challis, D. (1986) *Matching Resources to Needs in Community Care*. Aldershot: Gower.

Department of Health (1989) Caring for People: *Community Care in the Next Decade and Beyond*. (Cmd 849) London: HMSO.

Dincin, J., Wasner, D., Witheridge, T. F. (1993) Impact of assertive community treatment on the use of state hospital inpatient bed-days. *Hospital and Community Psychiatry*, 44, 833–838.

Dowson, S. (1990) 'Who does what? The Process of Enabling People with Learning Difficulties to Achieve What They Need and Want'. London: VIA.

Fisher, G. F., Landis, D., Clark, K (1988) Case management, service provision and client change. *Community Mental Health Journal*, 24(2), 134–142.

Franklin, J. L., Solovits, B., Mason, M., *et al.* (1994) An evaluation of case management. *American Journal of Public Health*, 77, 674–678.

Griffiths, R. (1988) *Community Care: Agenda for Action*. London: HMSO.

Harding, K., Baldwin, S., Baser, C. (1987) Towards multi-level needs assessments, *Behavioural Psychotherapy*, 15, 134–143.

Harris, M., Bergman, H. C. (1987) Case management with the chronically mentally ill: a clinical perspective. *American Journal of Orthopsychiatry*, 57, 296–302.

Holloway, F., McLean, E. K., Robertson, J. A. (1991). Case management. *British Journal of Psychiatry*, 159, 142–148.

Illich, I. (1977) *Disabling Professions*. London: Marion Boyars.

Intagliata, J. (1982) Improving the quality of community care for the chronically mentally disabled; the role of case management. *Schizophrenia Bulletin*, 8(4), 655–674.

Jenkins, J., Felce, D., Toogood, S., Mansell, J., de Kock, U. (1988) *Individual Programme Planning*. Kidderminster: BIMH Publications.

Marshall, M. (1995) Case management; a dubious practice. Under-evaluated and ineffective, but now government policy. *British Medical Journal*, 312, 523–524.

Marshall, M., Lockwood, A., Garth, D. (1995) Social services case management for long-term mental disorders: randomised controlled trial. *Lancet*, 345, 409–412.

Müeller, B. J., Hopp, M. (1987) Attitudinal, administrative, legal and fiscal barriers to case management in social rehabilitation of the mentally ill. *International Journal of Mental Health*, 15(4), 44–58.

Nadirshaw, Z. (1991) *Implications on the Assessment and Care Management of Black and Minority Ethnic People with Learning Difficulties and their Carers*. Occasional paper No. 2. London Boroughs Disability Resource Team.

Onyett, S. (1992) *Case Management in Mental Health*. London: Chapman and Hall.

Ovretveit, J. (1991) Case Management: notes for the perplexed. *Clinical Psychology Forum, Division of Clinical Psychology*, 36, October, 3–7.

Pilling, D. (1988) The Case Manager Project. *Re-Hab Network*, 10, 7–9.

Renshaw, J. (1988) Care in the community: individual care planning and case management. *British Journal of Social Work*, 10, 79–105.

Richardson, A., Higgins, R. (1990) *Case Management in Practice: Reflections on the Wakefield Case Management Project*. Working Paper 1. University of Leeds: Nuffield Institute for Health Service Studies.

Salisbury, B., Dickey, J., Crawford, C. (1987) *Service Brokerage: Individual Empowerment and Social Service Accountability*. Ontario: G Allan Roeher Institute.

Sevick, M. (1990) Case Management in University of Pittsburg. Unpublished PhD dissertation, University of Pittsburg, USA.

Shepherd, G. (1990) Case management. *Health Trends*, 22(2), 59–61.

Chapter 4

Needs assessment in a rehabilitation service

Karen Black

Service history

The population traditionally served by Airedale NHS Trust is mixed urban/rural, covering a large geographical spread of 560 square miles (1450 square kilometres). The psychiatric hospital that contained the rehabilitation and continuing-care beds was situated at the southern end of the catchment area. Services to the northern, more rural, part were less well developed.

When the decision to close the hospital was taken, it contained 102 rehabilitation and continuing-care beds. A rehabilitation service was in existence and community facilities, such as group homes, were in operation. However, recent changes in catchment areas meant that several group homes were physically in locations now served by a neighbouring service. Additionally, many people had been discharged from hospitals nearby into private accommodation and residential homes, within the boundaries. There was a rapidly changing set of circumstances and requirements. To develop community services (to facilitate the discharge and resettlement process) a multidisciplinary Community Rehabilitation/Resettlement Team was established. It was anticipated that as the team developed skills in community support, it would then establish a role as a specialist resource to other mental health teams and to other agencies, active in the locality.

The team was established to enable clients to develop the emotional, intellectual and physical skills needed to live, learn and work in their own environment. Efforts were focused on developing the clients' skills and resources to enable them to optimize their level of functioning. A large proportion of the work involved developing new community services to support the client and in coordinating existing services to ensure that clients are able to access and utilize them to their advantage.

Within the spirit of providing locally-based and easily accessible services, was supported a range of facilities including drop-in centres and day centres; individual and group-based support is also provided. To provide each client with access to all areas, agencies and resources, the team operates a specialist worker system. Individual members of the team work as specialists within different geographical locations. Consequently, the team has well-established links with a variety of other services, for example, community mental health centres (CMHCs), voluntary bodies, social services, charitable agencies in different parts of the district. In addition, it allows effective liaison and coordination of resources provided by these statutory and non-government agencies. This approach involves a single team with workers who develop detailed local knowledge and who liaise with other services and agencies. It recognizes the special and diverse difficulties experienced by individuals with enduring mental health problems. As the needs of the clients are complex and dynamic, it is essential that the service is able to isolate and identify separate needs, how they change and evaluate how far they are being met.

What are needs

Many different definitions of need exist. Kahn (1969), for example, emphasized their social nature, suggesting that needs are social definitions, representing a view of what an individual group requires in order to play a role, to meet a commitment or to participate adequately in a social process.

Bradshaw (1977), however, took a viewpoint that is more immediately recognizable to a clinician. He recognized four types of need: (i) normative need – that which an expert defines as need; (ii) felt need – consisting of input from an actual population as to what they feel they need; (iii) expressed need – a demand for service such as that reflected by waiting lists for services, and finally, (iv) comparative need – an inferred measure of need, determined by examining the characteristics of those people receiving services and then locating those characteristics in the population.

A more recent clarification (Brewin, 1992) is to characterize need in the following terms: (i) need is present when (a) a patient's functioning (social disablement) falls below or threatens to fall below some minimum specified level, and (b) this is due to a remediable, or potentially remediable cause; (ii) a need (as defined above) is met when it has attracted some at least partly effective item of care, and when no other items of care of greater potential effectiveness exist; (iii) a need (as defined above) is unmet when it has attracted only a partly effective solution.

The assessment of needs

Kimmel (1977) identified a range of one-dimensional techniques utilized in needs assessment. These range from the use of service statistics through problem incidence to the secondary analysis of opinion surveys. He concluded that, used in isolation, each of the techniques offers only a limited amount of data, and advocated the use of several such techniques in combination. Other approaches to needs assessment (Warheit et al., 1978) involve methods such as key informant, treatment rates and social indicators. The data collected by these techniques have invariably been used as an aid to service planning and resource allocation, rather than any clarification of the general or specific needs of individual clients (Steadman, 1980).

The significant limitation with these methods is that only a small proportion of the population under scrutiny is surveyed. Moreover, data utilizing key informants can result in erroneous conclusions, as respondents often have difficulty in identifying their problems or in expressing their needs.

A rehabilitation service, in addition to information about the individual needs of its clients, must also have an overview of the needs of its client group as a whole if services are to be planned and developed appropriately. The absence of objective data will create problems for service providers. Purchasers of health care will lack clear guidance when trying to exercise their responsibilities of allocating funds and resources appropriately.

Once needs have been successfully elicited from the population under scrutiny, how are the multitude of individual client needs to be ranked or collated to enable service priorities to be derived? One method might be to rank needs in terms of their intensity and prevalence within the given population (Murrell and Norris, 1983). Undoubtedly each client will regard each of their own needs to be important. Examination of the prevalence of any given need will not measure needs in terms of their importance to the client, but in terms of the number of clients who share that need. Services will be developed in terms of the commonality between clients. Potentially, this results in the creation of a highly restrictive set of services. Alternatively, the matter could be left to the judgement of the professionals/agencies involved in service delivery. Such an *ad hoc* arrangement would clearly create a situation in which the biases of the particular groupings and their ability to exert an influence over the system would determine which needs the service would attempt to meet.

The multi-level needs assessment

In the search for a needs assessment tool, it was clear that it should have a number of characteristics and serve a number of purposes. First, it must have the capability of not only identifying needs but also ranking these needs. Second, it should provide some indication of how well current resources meet client needs, along with clear indicators of how the organization or system is to meet identified needs.

A needs assessment instrument which was designed to measure needs at both individual and systemic levels is the *Multi-Level Needs Assessment* (MLNA) (Harding *et al.*, 1987). This instrument was designed in response to the move towards community care, in particular the desirability for any multi-level approach which focused on both the needs of consumers and workers. The sample utilized in the construction of the instrument comprised individuals in a variety of community settings (Part III accommodation, assessment unit, etc.) These individuals required considerable input from staff due to the problems they experienced as a result of some physical disability.

The instrument is divided into six main sections which the authors regarded as fundamental to a consideration of needs:

1 Interactions
2 Decisions and choices
3 What the person is like
4 Skills
5 Relationships
6 Events and experiences

Within each of these six sections are a number of subheadings. These contain specific questions which explore each area in more detail. Within the section Interactions, for example, the subheadings concern the areas of:

1 Communication
2 Adjustment
3 Physical health
4 Group membership
5 Self control

The assessment process requires the client's keyworker to work with the client in a close partnership, assessing needs, setting specific goals for intention and assessing the progress. The keyworker guides the client through the questions, exploring their needs and how each may be addressed by the service. Thus active individual programme planning takes place throughout the process.

The specific advantages of this highly-detailed process are, according to the authors, (a) its capacity to shape client and worker behaviour; (b) its capacity to shape care structures; (c) it provides meaningful records for both the client and worker; (d) it provides indicators for future service development.

The MLNA in practice

To establish the benefits of using the MLNA with the client group it was administered to a sample of 25 clients, selected as representative of the client group. The sample contained some clients who were relatively new to the service (less than one year) and some who had spent an extensive period (at least two years) with the team.

Using the MLNA to identify individual need

The following example indicates how the MLNA facilitated comprehensive and active individual programme planning.

Claire has been known to the service for 12 months. She had a long history of short admissions to hospital. Claire's family had, throughout the years, been supportive and had aided her integration back into her home environment. Claire's daily activities revolved around the home and her family. However, her family, while remaining supportive, had gradually moved away from the old family home and were no longer able to provide the previous levels of support. Her initial rehabilitation programme attempted to build adequate social networks which would offer Claire more immediate support and to provide her with opportunities for the development of interests and activities.

During her individual assessment Claire indicated that her existing programme had successfully enabled her to integrate back into her home environment. However, the assessment process gave clear indicators of the direction in which her programme needed to be developed. In particular, Claire highlighted areas concerning work. The MLNA thus enabled Claire to review her existing skills in relation to work and her preferences for work activity. After discussing in detail her skills and preferences, Claire was able to be steered into an appropriate work area. For the last three months Claire has worked in a local nursing home in a voluntary capacity. Both she and the manager of the nursing home are pleased with the progress she has made and are currently negotiating paid employment.

Using the MLNA to evaluate resources

As part of the assessment process, clients indicate the variety of resources they attend. From an analysis of the sample as a whole the popularity of each resource enabled an evaluation of the extent to which current resources are used and appreciated. The data suggested that resources initially created to afford clients the opportunities for socializing now appeared not to meet existing need. For example, within each locality drop-in facilities and day centres established by the team and by Social Services provided a social and activity centre. However, it appeared that the activities provided at these facilities were too general. Clients were asking for more specific group functions.

Particular issues identified by the process were that:

- Drop-ins in each geographical location appeared to possess a very unique identity.
- Group characteristics were variable in terms of age and gender bias.
- Activities offered were variable and seemed to be determined by the group facilitator rather than by clients.
- Geographical location hindered access, thereby impeding clients' ability to exercise choice by attending a facility most likely to meet their existing needs.

Using the MLNA to develop facilities and services

Following the analysis of client preferences, clients appeared to be asking for:

- Group-orientated activities.
- Opportunities for forming friendships.
- Community-based recreational activities.
- A broader access to facilities in terms of geographical location.
- Activities to take place out of normal working hours, in particular, more opportunity for attending groups in the evenings.
- Participation with others of a similar age range.

The above key indicators thus provided the impetus to review the structure and function of drop-in facilities. Following careful monitoring of attendance figures over a two-month period and following discussions with clients and drop-in facilitators, the decision was made to close one of them and to replace it with something designed more specifically to meet identified needs. The MLNA returns formed a blueprint for a replacement facility. The Social Activities Group (SAG) was designed.

Benefits of client choice

From its inception, the SAG quickly took on a very different identity to other facilities. The initial membership comprised clients between 20–30 years of age. It was intended that the group was to meet weekly. The location and the time of the group was flexible, being dependent on the particular activity. Trips were organized to sporting facilities, the theatre and the cinema. Shopping expeditions were held. While the team had, over the years, provided these activities, they had largely been dependent on the availability of staff and therefore took place on an *ad hoc* basis. The role of staff in the new group was low key: there was no need for direct facilitation but rather for someone who would take on the role of activity coordinator. Almost immediately the group became self-directing and activities were planned a month in advance. The group also decided to make a list of all forthcoming events and this was circulated to all clients on the team's caseload.

The membership of this group has grown over the months. Enquiries are now being received from other areas and agencies for clients who are not part of the team's caseload. The group is no longer restricted to the initial age range and the activities continue to be diverse. Clearly, the MLNA has enabled the creation of a facility which has become client-centred and self-perpetuating, rather than staff-centred and unpredictable. Moreover, keyworkers report individual benefits derived from group attendance. Friendships between clients have been the major benefit, resulting in the emergence of 'luncheon clubs'. In addition, many of the group activities have led to individual clients renewing their interest in hobbies. This suggests that empowering clients leads to changes which are more likely to be stable.

The use of the MLNA with complex cases

Many clients referred to the team have complex and multiple needs, for example behaviours such as self-harm and a history of physical violence and/or sexual abuse. These can occur within a context of psychiatric symptomatology. In order to address the diverse problems experienced by these clients the approach has been to introduce an associate worker alongside the keyworker. The keyworker coordinates all care, while the associate will be introduced to deal with one particular aspect of the client's problems. The following example attempts to make this clear.

Matching needs to helper skills

Kate had been attached to various mental health services for six years and many of her problems were related to her childhood abuse. Due to the sensitivity and the difficulties experienced by Kate, she had worked with various specialist health workers. Throughout the years prior to her referral to the rehabilitation team, Kate had many prolonged periods of hospital admission. These were invariably stormy times and discharge was fraught with difficulty. Staff doubted whether the admissions were really helpful. Following her MLNA, each of the areas Kate needed help with were identified. Kate was able to spell out clearly that when her situation became intolerable she regarded hospital admission as an essential component in her care. This gave subsequent admissions more focus and ward staff were able to see that Kate valued their intentions, although this was not always obvious at the time.

Kate reported that she found previous planned programmes of care confusing because one worker was attempting to deal with many separate issues all at once. Kate and her keyworker were thus able to identify her need for additional workers and those areas in which each worker could be involved. The MLNA clearly identified the need for three health professionals involved in Kate's care:

- One worker was to look specifically at the issues surrounding her abuse.
- One worker initially worked with Kate in the resettlement process and would continue increasing her social network thereby enabling Kate to integrate further into the community.
- One worker who coordinates her hospital admissions and deals with medication and monitoring issues.

In addition, a 'guesting' facility was incorporated into her programme in which she was able to come into hospital for a short period of respite care as opposed to admission.

The initial demands of this new programme plan were that workers had to adopt different working patterns. The worker coordinating hospital admission was designated as Kate's keyworker. The team member taking on this role would act as the focal point for all lines of communication with each of the other workers involved and for the service, thus ensuring that the response by each worker was fully coordinated and all approaches complementary. The worker dealing with the specific issue of abuse was co-opted from a Community Mental Health Centre in Kate's locality. This worker not only offered the essential expertise but also provided a resource more accessible in terms of geographical location for Kate. Consequently, while Kate was still able to discuss in detail all aspects of her care she now had clear boundaries as to the role of each worker; as a result sessions with her workers became more focused.

It was surprising that Kate wanted her care split in this way. Hitherto, it was assumed that it would be more appropriate to channel all care through one worker, who would build up a close supportive relationship with her. Listening to her, in the structured way that the MLNA requires, revealed that this was not her preference, and enabled staff to modify their input. This division of care would be quite inappropriate for other clients. The assessment process enabled the identification of Kate's preferred form of service delivery, and the necessary changes.

Since making these changes Kate has lived independently for over a year, which is the longest period of time she has survived in 'the community' for many years. Formal admissions due to medication misuse still occur, but they have shown a marked reduction in both frequency and duration. These formal admissions are interspersed with her use of the respite facility for periods of up to four days, after which she feels able to return home. Kate reports that this new method of working enables her to compartmentalize the different aspects of her life and she feels that she is making progress. In addition, workers report that this different working pattern allows them to share responsibility for her care and provides support for each worker.

Conclusions

The above findings are informal, in that they have been drawn from observation and have not been subjected to more rigorous evaluation. However, they clearly illustrate the utility of the MLNA. The MLNA offers a systematic needs assessment in which clients are actively involved in their programme planning. The assessment allows clients and their keyworkers to evaluate current programmes. Deficits in their care planning are identified and alternative plans of care can be constructed.

How often should the MLNA be repeated? Clients' needs are not fixed and they will change. The rate and extent of changes will be dependent on the variations in symptom severity, the occurrence of significant life changes and on many other external causes. The ultimate responsibility for the completion of the MLNA (according to Harding et al.) should remain with a named person; this is invariably the keyworker.

How much time does the assessment process take? The length and complexity of the assessment may prohibit the immediate completion of all sections. The assessment is constructed in such a way that several sections can be selected to start the needs assessment process; the remaining sections can be completed later. The general guide offered by the authors for the selection of sections is to target those areas more immediate to the person's needs (sections which are more important to the client). While the authors do not stipulate the frequency and duration of the assessment process, experience suggests that the process could be incorporated into current working practices in which the client and the keyworker dictate the frequency of the assessment. The potential limitation of the MLNA is that it relies extensively on the ability of clients to articulate their needs. While some clients are more capable of articulating their needs, it is unrealistic to expect all to be able to do so.

Within the sample Anna presented us with such a problem. Anna has spent a large proportion of her adult life within various institutional care settings. Communication with Anna is often difficult, her daily activities are severely limited. In line with the authors' suggestions, Anna was regarded as far as possible as the best source of information. The assessment proved to be long and difficult for both Anna and her keyworker. The authors suggest that relatives should be involved at this point to ascertain whether she had other ways of communicating how she manages. However, Anna has no living relatives. Various workers were then utilized as sources of information but each had diverging views of Anna's needs. However, after a long information gathering process, Anna's immediate need was her communication skills. After careful consideration of all possible interventions the goal was to utilize an advocate. The re-assessment of Anna's needs with her advocate is still pending.

Future plans

The aim is to use this method of assessment with all clients on the team's caseload. There is also a plan to introduce this assessment into the continuing-care facility. The continuing-care clients possess similar, but distinct patterns of disability. Due to the significant disabilities of this client group some difficulties are envisaged in using the MLNA as highlighted by Anna's assessment. Consequently the possibilities of introducing advocates are explored for some of the clients within this facility before the commencement of their assessment.

Active discussion in the non-government sector continues about the role of the MLNA in service development. The primary aim here would be to identify any duplication and omissions in the range of resources currently on offer by the team, other statutory services and the voluntary sector. In addition, the MLNA would allow an evaluation of the availability, accessibility, acceptability and patterns of use of service from all sectors. Full implementation of the assessment would involve the direct assessment of all clients using the voluntary sector. While this process would be feasible for those clients on the team's caseload, there is a high proportion of clients whose primary care is provided by other areas such as CMHCs. The next step may be to introduce the MLNA into these services. This would undoubtedly involve us in an intensive and time-consuming process.

While the above projects are in their infancy, we feel that appropriate use of the MLNA will enable the continuation of a client-focused service. The aim is to create a service that will undergo a continuous process of evolution and development in response to changing needs of clients, purchasers and providers of health care.

Acknowledgements

I would like to thank Dr Richard Shillitoe for his incisive comments and suggestions and also Catherine Thomas for her help in preparing earlier drafts of this chapter.

References

Bradshaw, J. (1977) The concept of social need. In *Planning for Social Welfare Issues, Models and Tasks* (N. Gilbert and H. Specht, eds). Englewood Cliffs, New Jersey: Prentice Hall.

Brewin, C. R. (1992) Measuring individual needs for care and services. In *Measuring Mental Health Needs* (G. Thornicroft, C. R. Brewin and J. Wing, eds). London: Gaskell.

Harding, K., Baldwin, S., Baser, C. *et al.* (1987) Towards multi-level needs assessment. *Behavioural Psychotherapy*, 15, 134–143.

Kahn, A. J. (1969) *Theory and Practice in Social Planning.* New York: Russell Sage Foundation.

Kimmel, W. A. (1977) *Needs Assessment: a Critical Perspective.* Office of Program Systems, OPS for Planning and Evaluation, Department of Health, Education and Welfare, Washington DC.

Murrell, S. A., Norris, T. H. (1983) Quality of life as the criterion for needs assessment and community psychology. *Journal of Community Psychology*, 11, 88–97.

Steadman, S. V. (1980) Learning to select a needs assessment strategy. *Training and Development Journal*, 56–61.

Warheit, G. J., Bell, R. A., Schwab, J. J. (1978) *Needs Assessment Approaches: Concepts and Methods.* US Department of Health Education and Welfare. Rockville, MD: NIMH.

Chapter 5

Assessing the needs of people who are disabled by serious ongoing mental health problems

Julie Repper and Rachel Perkins

Introduction

All current legislation relating to mental health invokes the concept of 'need' as a foundation for the development of services (DoH 1989, 1990, 1991, 1992, 1994). There is a lack of consistency and clarity in the way in which this concept is understood and put into operation. The theories and approaches considered are derived from those developed, practised and refined within two community-focused services for people who are disabled by serious ongoing mental health problems: the 'Rehabilitation and Community Care Service' of the Nottingham Healthcare Trust, and the 'Rehabilitation Services' of Pathfinder Mental Health Services NHS Trust in South London.

Defining the population

The way in which the population with serious ongoing mental health problems is defined is important in considering ideas about need. Some have suggested that psychiatric service contact should be the key variable. Shepherd (1984) for example, differentiated between old long-stay patients, new long-stay patients and new long-term patients:

Old long-stay patients are those people who have been hospitalized for many years, for whom the hospital has become 'home' and who have grown old there. This group of people often have a high level of physical health needs (Ford *et al.*, 1987). Many of their remaining problems are a consequence of institutionalization rather than the mental health difficulties that led to their original incarceration.

Typically they require a high level of support with day-to-day living, but display few disturbed and disturbing behaviours and are therefore relatively easy to help (Perkins *et al.*, 1989).

New long-term patients are those people who have developed ongoing mental health problems in a 'post-institutional' era and have not therefore been hospitalized for long periods. Although they often have extensive disabilities they have been supported by the various residential, day and outreach community services that have developed, as well as families and non-statutory agencies. Because they have not been chronically institutionalized, such people typically retain many normal expectations and skills. A lack of recognition of the extent of their disability is not uncommon among such people (Wing and Morris, 1981; Sheets *et al.*, 1982; Taylor and Perkins, 1991). Therefore they are often reluctant to use services unless particular care is taken to make support offered acceptable and accessible to them (Thompson, 1988; Repper and Perkins, 1994). This group needs support from services to decrease the impact of their disabilities upon the extent to which they can utilize their skills and realize their ambitions.

New long-stay patients are those people who have become long-term psychiatric inpatients in the 'post-institutional era'. Despite the community supports available, their disabilities and behaviour have been such that they cannot be accommodated outside a hospital-type setting (Shepherd, 1984). Clearly, the differentiation between 'new long-term' and 'new long-stay' clients cannot be based solely on characteristics of the clients themselves, but is equally a function of the nature and extent of community supports available. This group of people share many of the ordinary expectations and skills of their new long-term counterparts, but typically manifest a level of disturbed and disturbing behaviour that renders living in the community difficult for themselves and for those around them. The challenge for services is both to provide such people with the shelter they need and ensure that they retain skills and community contacts to prevent them suffering the consequences of institutionalization that so disable their old long-stay counterparts.

Despite the utility of such a 'service usage' typology in clinical practice, it is fraught with difficulties; it does not include the many people with serious problems who have never entered services or who drop out, returning only infrequently (and often involuntarily) at times of crisis. In a critical review of definitions of people with serious ongoing mental health problems, Bachrach (1988) identified three dimensions on which the population has been defined: diagnosis, duration and disability.

Serious mental health problems are often considered synonymous with a diagnosis of schizophrenia, or at the very most, with one of psychosis. Although those with such diagnoses form the bulk of long-term populations (Shepherd, 1988), even a cursory look at such populations using services reveals a plethora of diagnoses, ranging from Huntington's chorea and Korsakoff psychosis to personality disorder and various anxiety-based problems (people with extensive disabilities are very difficult to classify within diagnostic systems) (Perkins and Greville, 1993). To consider only a circumscribed range of diagnoses means that the needs of many people will not be addressed, and they are effectively denied the services they require. Concerns about such people 'falling through the net' are rife (Hirsch *et al.*, 1992).

Definitions based on duration are typically based on length of service contact, but there is no necessary relationship between duration of such contact and need. This effectively ignores the needs of three groups: those people who have extensive disabilities but have not yet had them for a sufficiently long period to meet duration criteria; people who 'drop in and out' and therefore fail to meet any duration criteria that requires a period of continuous contact; and the many people who have ongoing mental health problems in the homelessness and criminal justice system and who never enter psychiatric services (Timms and Fry, 1989; Weller, 1989).

Probably the most useful approach to defining the population is through a model of disability, and in particular social disability, (the extent to which the person is able to perform socially to the standards they expect of themselves, that others expect of them, or that society in general expects) (Wing and Morris, 1981; Shepherd, 1984). Such a conceptualization has the advantage of considering not only the individual, but their social context and relationships. Neither disability nor need can be defined in a vacuum; they can only be assessed in relation to the social world in which the person functions and the expectations of that world. By definition, everyone who comes into contact with psychiatric services has failed in some way to meet such expectations, therefore their 'needs' must be understood in terms of meeting the demands placed upon them.

If the person has ongoing disabilities as a consequence of their mental health problems, then they may not be able to change to 'fit in' to the world around them. As with physical disability, ensuring access to the society that they need involves changing the world to fit the individual as much, if not more, than helping the individual to change to fit the world (Perkins and Dilks, 1992; Kitzinger and Perkins, 1993; Repper and Perkins, 1996; Perkins and Repper, 1996). The consideration of 'needs' presented in this chapter is therefore based on the following premises:

1 The population with serious ongoing mental health problems can most usefully be defined in terms of the disability attendant on such problems, rather than the diagnosis they have been accorded, or the duration of their contact with services.
2 People with such problems might best be considered 'socially disabled' – unable to perform on a day-to-day basis to the standards expected in the communities within which they live.
3 The aim of services and supports should be to ensure access to social roles, activities and facilities for those people who are socially disabled in much the same way as ensuring access to the physical world for people who are physically disabled.
4 Ensuring access, whether it be to the social or physical world, involves changing those worlds to accommodate the individual (by providing the necessary supports, shelter and adaptations) as much, if not more, than changing the individual him/herself.
5 Any assessment of 'need' within this context must therefore involve both an assessment of the individual and the social environment in which they function (or wish to function).

Defining needs in relation to social access

If needs assessment is construed in these terms, then numerous difficulties arise concerning what is a need and who should define it. The term 'need' has been used to refer to everything from 'basic' bodily needs such as nutrition and warmth, through to emotional needs, and there are many 'interested parties' with quite different agendas competing for the right to specify these needs. Of central importance, there is the individual him/herself who has views about what his/her needs are. There are also mental health professionals, families, friends and relatives, the police, other agencies in the community. These exist within a general social context in which certain needs are culturally or temporally deemed more important than others. Too often, it is assumed that a consensus between all of these groups can be reached but their priorities are often quite different. In general, there is a distinction between three perspectives: a 'civil rights' approach which accords pride of place to the individual's right to choose; a 'duty of care' approach which emphasizes the need to protect vulnerable individuals (often from themselves) and make decisions for those people who may not always appear able to make decisions for themselves; and a 'law and order' approach which prioritizes the need to keep communities free from disturbed and disturbing individuals who might be disruptive to the lives of other citizens.

It is not the focus of this chapter to consider these approaches in detail, but it is important to recognize that the needs defined within each framework will differ. For example, a 'law and order' approach might focus on disruptive behaviour in assessing need, while a 'duty of care' model might emphasize vulnerability to harm and risk, and a 'civil rights' perspective would be primarily concerned with the wants and wishes of the disabled individual and the impediments to achieving their ambitions.

Any definition of need inevitably involves political and ethical judgements. Within the limitations of the legislative framework that pertains – most notably the 1983 Mental Health Act – the present discussion will adopt a 'civil rights' perspective. Wherever possible primacy is accorded to the wants and wishes of the individual and facilitating their access to the roles and lives they wish to lead. In doing so it is not possible to ignore the views of others (friends, relatives, neighbours). Their ability to accommodate the individual is an important part of that person gaining access to the social world. It is often the case that either the views and behaviours of others must be changed to allow access for the disabled person, or the person themselves must change to be acceptable.

The needs of people disabled by serious mental health problems

People with social disabilities as a result of serious mental health problems have the same human needs as the rest of the population. Any differences lie not in needs, but in terms of the personal, social and material resources available to meet those needs (Perkins and Dilks, 1992; Repper and Perkins, 1994b, 1996; Perkins and Repper, 1996). In a recent survey in the USA (Estroff, 1993) people with serious ongoing mental health problems defined their most frequently unmet needs to be in the areas of: an adequate income; a satisfying sexual life; meaningful work; a satisfying social life; happiness; adequate resources; warmth and intimacy; privacy. Although these are patently all basic needs with which anyone might identify, they are broad and general areas which do not reflect individual differences in life experiences and expectations. For example, a need for a satisfying sex life means different things to a lesbian woman and a heterosexual man; warmth and intimacy might conjure different pictures, and hence require different forms of help for people in different age groups, of different sex, from different cultures and ethnic groups.

It is essential that the special needs of different individuals and minority groups are not overlooked. Bachrach (1985) suggests that women with chronic mental illness are 'doubly disadvantaged', first by being 'mentally ill' [sic] and second by being female. The same might be said for all people who belong to the many possible minority groups. Services are frequently planned and provided by white, middle class heterosexual men with the most demanding (in terms of numbers and behaviour) client group in mind: young men with a diagnosis of schizophrenia. Thus, while buildings, services, organizational systems and individual interventions purport to serve a whole population, they often implicitly and unintentionally discriminate against people with special or different needs. It is the responsibility of health care workers actively to observe, attend, listen and ask, in order to assess and meet the particular needs of every individual; it cannot be assumed that the ordinary routine, meals, sanitary provision, religious pictures on the walls, even language will meet the needs of all people using the service. To avoid irritating and unnecessary questions or blunders, there should be a level of awareness among staff about the needs of particular groups of people through regular teaching, up-dating and access to specific information. Further, since dietary needs, translated information and spiritual needs will be required regularly by people in particular groups, access to such provision should be agreed on a long-term basis.

While it is essential not to put all people with serious ongoing mental health problems into one generic group, it is also important not to define the needs of these people in terms of the services that are available. All too often, mental health professionals define someone as 'needing a day centre' or 'needing a hostel'. No one 'needs' a day centre or a hostel; these are just one way of providing the support and shelter that a person requires. It is not enough to rely on the division frequently made between 'service led' and 'needs driven' models as the critical issue in the way in which 'needs' are defined. A 'needs driven' model can in effect be identical to a 'service led' model if needs are defined in terms of services: if a person is defined as needing a hostel because they cannot budget and bathe unaided, then this 'needs driven' approach is essentially service led.

A further problem with defining needs in terms of their solutions (a day centre or hostel) is that it detracts from the range of options that may be available in meeting a person's needs – and different options may be more acceptable to different people. Further, service solutions such as day centres and hostels can result in the undesirable institutional practice of 'block treatment'. Because they serve a range of individuals, with a commensurate range of problems and needs, such care cannot readily be tailored to any one person, often resulting in over-provision and detracting from the unique pattern of interests, abilities and problems each person may have.

People with serious ongoing mental health problems are multiply, but not universally, disabled. That is, they may have problems in several areas (for example they may have difficulty making and sustaining new relationships, their flat may be unsuitable and they cannot keep it as clean as they would like, and they may have great difficulty coping with letters, bills and money), but they also have skills and strengths in other areas (for example, the same person may be totally reliable about visiting his mother weekly and may have a well-maintained collection of stamps). Therefore any assessment of need must focus not only on what a person cannot do, but what they can and want to do. Thus it becomes clear what needs to be done in order to create opportunities for using strengths and pursuing interests. In recent years there has been a move away from traditional problem-based needs assessment towards a strengths approach which focuses at least as much on what the person can do and wants to do as on their cognitive, emotional and behavioural limitations.

Before proceeding to consider a strengths approach to needs assessment (Kirstardt and Rapp, 1989) in more detail, there is one further feature of needs that is important. In traditional models, especially those within the fields of physical and learning disabilities, it is assumed that a person's disabilities are relatively stable. Therefore the assumption is that people are helped to reach their optimal level of functioning and a network of aids and supports organized to enable them to stay there. Unfortunately, serious ongoing mental health problems are not like this. People with such problems are particularly vulnerable to social stressors and even relatively minor upsets and life events can increase cognitive, emotional and behavioural difficulties (Ambelas, 1979, 1987; Day et al., 1987; Birley, 1991). Thus the needs of an individual can vary widely over very short periods of time, and a simple linear progression or improvement cannot be assumed. Consequently, needs assessment is something that must be repeated not only on a regular basis, but also flexibly in response to changes in the person and their situation.

Why assess needs?

In any assessment, the reasons for that assessment determine the methods that will be appropriate. In relation to people with serious ongoing mental health problems there are three main reasons why needs might be assessed:

The planning and design of services

For these purposes, details of individual needs are not required. Instead, a more 'broad brush' approach is necessary to ensure that an adequate range of structures exists to serve the needs of individuals in the target population. Consequently, the numbers of people requiring different categories of support need are required.

The assessment of change over time

At a population level, similar data to that described above are necessary, but it may also be important to evaluate the change in individuals over time (e.g. to assess the effectiveness of the services provided in meeting needs). There are numerous parameters on which such change might be evaluated, but all require some assessment that produces numerical indices: assessing change in verbal descriptions is almost impossible. Useful areas to assess and assessment tools might include:

- Social functioning, e.g. REHAB assessment (Hall and Baker, 1983), Life Skills Profile (Rosen et al., 1989), Social Behaviour Schedule

(Wykes and Sturt, 1988).
- Psychiatric symptomatology, e.g. Brief Psychiatric Rating Scale (Overall and Gorham, 1962), Krawieka, Goldberg and Vaughn Scale (Krawieka *et al.*, 1977).
- Quality of life, e.g. Quality of Life Interview (Lehman, 1983; Simpson *et al.*, 1989).
- Social networks, e.g. Social Network Assessment (TAPS), Inventory of Socially Supportive Behaviours (Barrera, 1978).

Planning the support and care of the individual

In this context a detailed understanding of all facets of the person and their situation is required. While standard assessments such as those listed above may have some utility in identifying individual needs in this regard, they offer insufficient detail regarding each individual to be sufficient on their own. Further, they offer extremely sparse information about the social context in which the person functions and the problems and possibilities this affords. The remainder of this chapter will be concerned with needs assessment in relation to planning help for individuals who experience serious ongoing mental health problems.

The strengths approach

The strengths model outlined by Kirstardt and Rapp (1989) is essentially an approach to the whole of care planning and delivery, not simply to needs assessment. However, three of the principles on which it is founded are of central importance to the needs assessment process.

The focus is on individual strengths rather than on pathology

Anyone prefers to spend time doing things that they like, do well, and which have meaning for them. People with serious ongoing mental health problems are no different. Development, growth and a satisfying life are dependent on the extent to which a person can pursue their interests, aspirations and strengths. It is therefore critical that any needs assessment focuses on an assessment of the person's strengths and aspirations – the things they can do, as well as those they cannot. Without such assessment there is no way in which care can be planned to enable the person to exploit their strengths and pursue their interests.

In addition, services often have difficulty in 'engaging' clients (Repper and Perkins, 1994b). Such engagement problems often result from the person seeing the services that they are offered as irrelevant to their wants and needs. If the care and support offered is based on an assessment of strengths, wishes and aspirations, then the person is more likely to take up the option.

The community is viewed as an 'oasis of opportunity' rather than as an obstacle

Historically, little attention was paid to the environment in which the person functioned: all their difficulties were attributed to their individual pathology. Early considerations of 'the community' tended to emphasize the problems posed for the disabled individual: the stigma and day-to-day difficulties of living outside a sheltered environment (e.g. Wing and Morris, 1981). Such a conceptualization has led to a tendency to provide little segregated lacunae in the community (like day centres and hostels) where the person can gain relief from the stresses of community life. In contrast, a strengths approach emphasizes the opportunities that the community already offers and ways in which these can be extended and enhanced.

Any community offers a far greater range of opportunities than a segregated psychiatric service could ever provide. For needs assessment, the focus is upon access to these opportunities. Such an assessment might incorporate an exploration of support that could be provided and ways in which the existing facilities might be changed, to accommodate the individual, as well as ways the individual might change.

Interventions are based on the client's wants and wishes

Thus any assessment of need must take as its central focus the wants and wishes of the individual him or herself. Sometimes a person is not able to identify their wants and aspirations, in which case a major need is to help them to work out what it is they want. More often professionals assert that their clients' aspirations are 'unrealistic', (for example when clients say that they want to get married and have a job, children and a home of their own, all of which would be very ordinary for someone not defined as a 'psychiatric patient'). However, if clients' aspirations are accepted, then it is possible to negotiate the steps towards helping them to achieve their goals.

For example, if the client wants to be a nurse then they will need to have a nursing qualification; to get on to a nursing course they will need secondary school qualifications; to get these they will need to read and write; to do this they will need to go to college; to do this they will need to get up in the morning, dress appropriately, get the college prospectus, get to the college to register and turn up regularly ... These are all 'needs' that the client has for their own stated goal. A plan can then be constructed to help clients achieve these, providing the necessary support along the way (for example someone to help them obtain the prospectus or get up in the morning). Some people will discover the targets they have set themselves are too high (everyone comes to this realization at times), but this does not invalidate the effort of helping clients get as far as they can, nor does it decrease the value of achievements made along the way. The person may never get a nursing qualification, but every step is of value. As the person progresses, so their needs, wants and aspirations change, so assessment must be ongoing: no needs assessment is ever a 'once and for all' event.

What to assess

Typically, needs assessment schedules employed in services for people with serious ongoing mental health problems consist of various 'checklists' to direct the assessor towards exploring different areas of the person's functioning and experience. Many such schedules have been developed, which adopt slightly different approaches. The purpose of this account is not to define a 'blueprint', but to consider the areas that must be covered if the assessment is adequately to address the multiplicity of needs of people with serious ongoing mental health problems. Only the broad areas of assessment are outlined; specific questions are influenced by the individuals concerned. The approach which, in this account, lies within the framework of social disability, access and strengths outlined above also should be considered.

Personal, social, work and family history

The past of many people with ongoing mental health problems has been lost in the mists of time. Psychiatric notes often contain copious detail on the person's progress within psychiatric services – the history of their identity as 'patient' – but little (if anything) about what else they are, or have been. If the person is to have access to the ordinary social world, if their strengths, wants, hopes and fears are to be recognized, the first task of any needs assessment must be to discover the person apart from their illness, the numerous identities they may have had (mother, worker, saxophone player, undergraduate, cat lover), the interests that may have fuelled these endeavours, the skills associated with them, and the social, political and family context within which they occurred.

Psychiatric service and treatment history

Although people with serious and ongoing mental health problems have often been hospitalized for many years, often there is little accessible information about the treatments, interventions and supports provided during this time and the success or otherwise of these. Daunted by numerous thick volumes of illegible notes, it is not unusual for health care staff to remain unaware of what a client's experiences of services has been. Consequently, opportunities are missed to build upon successes of the past, avoid previous mistakes and understand clients' attitudes towards the help that is offered. A person's experience of psychiatric services is often a prominent feature of their life and therefore forms an important context for understanding their current needs; no-one should be a prisoner of their past, however. People can and do change, things that did not 'work' in the past may 'work' now.

A consideration of an individual's history both within and outside psychiatric services has an additional function in meeting the needs of staff who might be working with them. Staff frequently find work with severely disabled clients difficult and demoralizing. However, knowing the person's experiences both within (and outside) services can enable staff to understand better the origins of, and reasons for, behaviours they find difficult, to enable them to understand such responses more effectively, and tolerate them more easily.

The individual and their environment

The final aspect of a needs assessment comprises a thorough assessment of the individual and his/her environment. The numerous areas to include cannot be covered through a single interview; there must be time to help each individual explore and develop their ideas, views and priorities regarding their current problems, strengths and interests in all areas of their life, the things they would like to achieve, their ambitions in relation to such things as living arrangements, social relationships, work and leisure, their views of the help that they are currently receiving and have received in the past. It is also important to assess the things that they would like help with, what sort of help, how and from whom; if a person is given the help they want in the way that they want it, they are much more likely to accept it.

It is essential that a thorough assessment of their strengths and problems in all areas of functioning is also conducted. This will include: physical health, personal hygiene and domestic chores, work/employment, leisure, social contacts, family and social relationships, financial and legal concerns and accommodation. A full assessment of their mental health is also important, including their usual symptoms, how they feel about these, what helps or hinders symptomatology, prodromal signs, the effectiveness of medication, knowledge about medication, control of medication and side effects of medication.

Although symptoms are often the reason for initial contact with psychiatric services, it is likely that these no longer take precedence over the difficulties that people experience in practical or social domains. Details of how to assess symptomatology, what to assess, and why, are given in various mental health or psychiatric texts. Mental health should be considered in terms of the effects that it has on the person's everyday life, and the effects that everyday life has on the person's symptoms.

Finally it is essential that the individual's social network is assessed to monitor whom they see, for what purpose and how they get on. Although supportive relationships have been found to be protective in terms of initial breakdown, people with serious ongoing mental health problems are particularly sensitive to stressors, particularly within close and continuing relationships such as families. There is now evidence from a variety of sources that the level of 'expressed emotion' within families can profoundly influence the functioning of the disabled individual and determine the extent to which they have access to such relationships (Brown et al., 1972; Vaughn and Leff, 1976; Brooker et al., 1991). Needs assessment should include an evaluation of family relationships and coping, so that appropriate remedial action can be taken.

Having gained a full picture of the person, their views about what they want and how it should be offered, their problems and strengths need to be listed and priorities accorded. A strengths-based approach requires a consideration of all areas in relation to the client's circumstances and what they wish to achieve. A skills deficit is only a problem if it prevents the person from achieving something that they want to achieve. For example, if someone cannot cook this may or may not be a problem. If a woman wishes to have children, the cooking may well be necessary, but if she has no aspirations in this direction then she could easily make use of take-aways and cafes (as many people do) rather than cook. Often services staff make the mistake of focusing on the 'basics' of life at the expense of consideration of the context of the person's skills. Self-care and domestic activities often receive inappropriate priority over leisure, work and social activities. If such activities are unimportant to clients, then continued emphasis on such areas is likely both to alienate clients and to fail to maximize the skills they do have.

If a person is severely socially disabled they may be unable to do all that is expected of them; sometimes it is necessary to relieve them of certain tasks and roles in order to facilitate engagement in others. Most people would agree that it is more important to their sense of value and esteem to engage in work, leisure and social activities rather than to wash their socks. Although there will be many individual differences in this regard, clients are likely to share this perception. In terms of the environment in which the person functions, it is important to consider the naturally occurring supports and services that might be employed in two ways. First, resources should be identified which enable the client to gain access to the roles, relationships, facilities and activities they desire. Second, those facilities should be identified which might be employed to minimize the disruptive impact of any disabilities and problems they might have. This might include family, friends, neighbours, non-psychiatric services, churches, self-help groups, the availability of service washes in launderettes, cheap cafes and take-aways, as well as the 'psychiatric services' on which mental health professionals too frequently focus.

It is not enough merely to find out about these resources and send the client along. The characteristics of the facilities must be considered if they are to provide effective support for the disabled individual. This might include anything from respite arrangements for families, to easily accessible help in emergencies, education and information, and ongoing support from psychiatric services – anything that will increase the accessibility of the community for the individual with social disabilities.

To enable any individual to maximize their potential, it is essential to identify those aspects of the environment which exacerbate their problems and which prevent them from exploiting their abilities and realizing their ambitions. Although communities can be an oasis of possibility, they can also be stigmatizing: the consequences of negative attitudes can deny access to people who appear 'odd' to numerous facilities and activities. An important aspect of needs assessment is the identification of what would be required to decrease such discrimination. It is important not to forget the disabling effects of being within psychiatric services. The negative consequences of hospitalization are well documented (Barton, 1959; Goffman, 1961; Wing and Brown, 1961), but many of the community services also have their problems. For example, it is difficult to entertain friends or family in many residential facilities which might make relationships difficult to sustain. Living in shared accommodation with people not of one's choosing is stressful for anyone, and people with ongoing mental health problems are particularly vulnerable to such stressors. Equally, the stigmatizing effects of collecting psychotropic medication from a chemist, or walking into a mental health clinic, should be recognized.

Conclusion: disability, access and opportunity

Needs assessment can never be an 'objective' exercise, it is essentially based on the context and purpose of the needs assessment, the way in which needs are conceptualized, and the theoretical framework adopted. The difficulties facing someone with serious ongoing mental health problems might best be understood as social disabilities, which impede the individual's functioning in the ordinary ('able-minded') social world in much the same way as physical limitations impede functioning in the ordinary (able-bodied) physical world. In the conceptualization offered here, the aims of intervention are to ensure that the socially disabled person has access to the ordinary social world, just as the physically disabled person has access to the physical world.

If the disabilities of a person who experiences serious ongoing mental health problems were conceptualized within an entirely organic model, then a very different assessment of needs would be presented. The aim would be to reduce symptoms to a minimum (if not to eliminate them) and all interventions would be judged in terms of their ability to achieve this. In contrast, it is suggested here that symptoms are not unimportant, but only one of many factors that prevent such access. Clearly, one might want to reduce the person's cognitive and emotional problems, but this is not the overriding aim. Often a level of medication that minimizes symptomatology is not commensurate with optimal functioning and access – high levels of medication can leave the person tired, lethargic, and with adverse side effects, all of which detract from their ability to perform everyday activities.

This approach to needs assessment is predicated on the assumption that the aim is not necessarily to get rid of a person's symptoms and problems, but (in line with a strengths approach) to minimize the destructive consequences of disabilities, and maximize a person's access to the opportunities that everyone else enjoys: to enable them to pursue their aspirations and goals despite their disabilities.

References

Ambelas, A. (1979) Psychological stressful events in the precipitation of manic episodes. *British Journal of Psychiatry*, **135**, 15–21.

Ambelas, A. (1987) Life events and mania: a special relationship? *British Journal of Psychiatry*, **150**, 235–240.

Bachrach, L. L. (1985) Chronically mentally ill women: emergence and legitimation. *Hospital and Community Psychiatry*, **36**, 1063–1069.

Bachrach, L. L. (1988) Defining mental illness: a concept paper. *Hospital and Community Psychiatry*, **38**, 383–388.

Barrera, M. (1978) A method for the assessment of social support networks in community survey research. *Connections*, **3**, 8–15.

Barton, R. (1959) *Institutional Neurosis*. Bristol: Wright.

Brooker, C., Butterworth, C., Tarrier, N., Barrowclough, C. (1992) Training community psychiatric nurses to undertake psychosocial intervention: changes in role. *International Journal of Nursing Studies*, **28**, 189–200.

Birley, J. (1992) Schizophrenia: the problems of handicap. In *Community Psychiatry* (D. Bennett and H. Freeman, eds). London: Churchill Livingstone.

Brown, G. W., Birley, J. L. T., Wing, J. K. (1972) Influence of family life on the course of schizophrenic disorders: a replication. *British Journal of Psychiatry*, **121**, 241–258.

Day, R., Neilson, J. A., Korten, A. (1987) Stressful life events preceding the acute onset of schizophrenia: a cross national study from the World Health Organization. *Culture, Medicine and Society*, **11**, 123–205.

DoH (1989) *Caring for People. Community Care into the Next Decade and Beyond*. London: HMSO.

DoH (1990) *NHS and Community Care Act*. London: HMSO.

DoH (1991) *Implementing Community Care*. London: HMSO.

DoH (1992) *Health of the Nation*. London: HMSO.

DoH (1994) *Working in Partnership*. London: HMSO.

Estroff, S. (1983) Community Mental Health Services: Extinct, Endangered or Evolving? Paper presented at conference Mental Health Practice in the Nineties: Changes and Challenges. Silver Springs, MD.

Ford, M., Goddard, C., Lansdallwelfare, R. (1987) The dismantling of the mental hospital? Glenside Hospital Surveys 1960–1985. *British Journal of Psychiatry* 151, 479–485.

Goffman, E. (1961) *Asylums*. Harmondsworth: Pelican.

Hall, J. N., Baker, R. (1983) *Users Manual of Rehabilitation Evaluation Hall and Baker (REHAB) Scale*. Aberdeen: Vine Publishing.

Hirsch, S., Craig, T., Dean, C., Hollander D., Holloway, F., Howat, J., et al. (1992) *Facilities and Services for the Mentally Ill with Persisting Severe Disabilities*. Working Party Report on Behalf of the Royal College of Psychiatrists.

Kirstardt, W. E., Rapp, C. A. (1989) *Bridging the Gap between Principles and Practice. Implementing a Strengths Perspective in Case Management*. Kansas City: The University of Kansas Press.

Kitzinger, C., Perkins, R. E. (1993) *Changing our Minds: Lesbian Feminism and Psychology*. London: Only Women Press.

Krawieka, M., Goldberg, D., Vaughan, M. (1977) A standardised psychiatric assessment scale for rating chronic psychotic patients. *Acta Psychiatrica Scandinavica*, 55, 299–308.

Lehman, A. F. (1983) The well-being of chronic mental patients: assessing their quality of life. *Archives of General Psychiatry*, 40, 369–373.

Overall, J. E., Gorham, D. R. (1962) The brief psychiatric rating scale. *Psychological Medicine*, 10, 799–812.

Perkins, R. E., King, S., Hollyman, J. A. (1989) Resettlement of old long-stay psychiatric patients: the use of the private sector. *British Journal of Psychiatry*, 155, 233–238.

Perkins, R. E., Dilks, S. (1992) Worlds apart. Working with severely socially disabled people. *Journal of Mental Health*, 1, 3–17.

Perkins, R. E., Greville L. (1993) *Long Term Case Register: Fourth Annual Report*. London: Wandsworth Health Authority.

Perkins, R., Repper, J. (1996) *Working Alongside People with Long Term Mental Health Problems*. London: Chapman and Hall.

Repper, J., Perkins, R. (1994a) The deserving and the undeserving: selectivity and progress in a community service. *Journal of Mental Health*, 8, 483–498.

Repper, J., Perkins, R. (1994b) Meeting the needs of neglected patients. *Nursing Standards*, 9(2), 28–31.

Rosen, A., Hadzi-Pavlovic, D., Parker, G. (1989) The life skills profile: a measure assessing function and disability in schizophrenia. *Schizophrenia Bulletin*, 15, 325–337.

Sheets, J. L., Prevost, J. A., Reihman, J. (1982) Young adult chronic patients: three hypothesised sub-groups. *Hospital and Community Psychiatry*, 3, 197–202.

Shepherd, G. (1984) *Institutional Care and Rehabilitation*. New York: Longman.

Shepherd, G. (1988) Current Issues in Community Care. Report on the 2nd

Annual Conference on the Rehabilitation of Psychiatric Patients and their Care in the Community, 13.12.88. The Association of Psychological Therapies.

Simpson, C. J., Hyde, C. E., Faragher, E. B. (1989) The chronically mentally ill in community facilities: a study of quality of life. *British Journal of Psychiatry*, **154**, 77–82.

Taylor, K. E., Perkins, R. E. (1991) Identity and coping with mental illness in long-stay rehabilitation. *British Journal of Clinical Psychology*, **30**, 73–85.

Thompson, E. H. (1988) Variation in the self-concept of young adult chronic patients: youthful chronicity re-considered. *Hospital and Community Psychiatry*, **39**, 260–264.

Timms, P. W., Fry, A. H. (1989) Homelessness and mental illness. *Health Trends*, **21**, 71–72.

Vaughn, C., Leff, J. (1976) The influence of family and social factors on the course of psychiatric illness. *British Journal of Psychiatry*, **129**, 125–137.

Weller, M. (1989) Psychosis and destitution at Christmas 1985–1988. *Lancet*, ii, 1509–1511.

Wing, J. K., Brown, G. W. (1961) *Institutionalisation and Schizophrenia*. Cambridge: Cambridge University Press.

Wing, J. K., Morris, B. (1981) Clinical basis of rehabilitation. In *Handbook of Psychiatric Rehabilitation Practice* (J. K. Wing, ed.) Oxford: Oxford University Press.

Wykes, T., Sturt, D. (1986) The measurement of social behaviours in psychiatric patients: an assessment of the reliability and validity of the SBS schedule. *British Journal of Psychiatry*, **148**, 1–11.

Chapter 6

Needs assessment in elderly people suffering from communication difficulties and/or cognitive impairment

Ingalill Rahm Hallberg

Introduction

The increasing number of old people, especially very old elderly, puts more and more demands on society for high quality and cost-effective care. This development goes for Sweden, Europe, and the rest of the world (The National Board of Health and Welfare, 1993). Naturally the elderly person's self-care abilities shrink and he or she becomes increasingly dependent on others for fulfilling needs. Complementary care is required and it may be provided by a next of kin or by a formal caregiver. The care may be provided in institutional settings of various types or in the elderly person's home. In spite of where and who is providing the care it needs to be based on a thorough assessment of the care recipient's needs.

Needs assessment as a basis for the framework and provision of care is especially demanding when it concerns elderly people with communication or cognitive deficits. These people often cannot easily speak for themselves either in terms of current problems, likes or dislikes or of how they want the help to be performed. This problem affects people suffering from congenital or degenerative cognitive impairment and dysphasia and especially those suffering from dementia disorders of various types (McLean, 1987a,b). The communication difficulties mean that they cannot easily participate in a cooperative delineation of their care needs. This problem may also affect people with psychomotor latency, for instance elderly and depressed people (Heston *et al.*, 1992). They may have problems formulating their ideas at a speed that accords with the caregiver's work pace and patience.

The problem of mutual cooperation in assessing the care recipient's needs and the fact that the caregiver and the care recipient cannot reach consensus on what the care should focus, increases with the complexity of the recipient's deficits. For instance, in the case of dementia, the person suffers from communication problems of an impressive as well as expressive type (Wallin *et al.*, 1994). They also suffer from cognitive impairment, making it difficult for them to organize, for instance, perceptions, feelings and previous experiences into a meaningful whole. It is even more difficult to transfer this to another person. The fact that the person cannot cognitively organize impressions into an understandable whole does not mean that the person does not feel and react to situations. This picture is complicated even more by the fact that people suffering from dementia become successively more dependent on the caregivers to fulfil all their basic needs (McLean, 1987a,b). The care recipient has a great need for supplementary care. This means that the caregiver has to override the person's intimate boundaries and perhaps even 'intrude' into the most intimate zones in order to provide the necessary care. The care recipient sometimes reacts to these caring actions with anger and frustration (Hallberg *et al.*, 1995). This may be their way of validating the nurse's interpretation of his or her needs. Thus poorly adapted care may explain that much resistance, force and the use of power over one another tend to be inherent in care of the demented people (Hallberg *et al.*, 1995).

The needs assessment of an elderly care recipient must be based on a broad and dynamic model for assessing and interpreting the needs of the individual. Attempts have been made to define and clarify the concept of needs assessment (McWalter *et al.*, 1994), but such definitions may entail the risk of reducing needs assessment when applied in practice. Needs assessment can be instrumental for bringing into focus peoples' difficulties in fulfilling their basic physical and psychosocial needs (Maslow, 1954). For that purpose various assessment tools and measures can be used to show that all people are assessed in a reliable and valid manner. The problems with such an approach are that the assessment (e.g. of cognitive decline or reduced functional ability) cannot easily be translated into needs that have been assessed.

Keywords for a focus in the needs assessment can be used to guide the assessment (like in the Swedish VIPS-system: Well-being, Integrity, Prevention, Safety) (Ehnfors *et al.*, 1991). The assessment can also be based on the idea that the goal of care is to support or take over the care recipient's maintenance of important values and goals in his or her everyday life; prevention of any unnecessary hurt or injury to the person in the provision of care should be paramount. Needs assessment must investigate the gap between the care recipients' view of the important values and goals in life and the deficiencies that hinder them from maintaining these aspects in their everyday life. Account should be made of what may hurt them, or exceed their capacity. Even such a framework for needs assessment means excluding important aspects that shape the care recipients' current needs.

The care recipient is a victim of the environment

It has been hypothesized that the more dependent and impaired a person is, the fewer resources he or she has for adapting the environment to basic needs or for adapting to the environment (Lawton, 1980; Svensson, 1984). Thus s/he is a victim of environmental conditions. In addition, the more poorly adapted the environmental conditions are to the care recipient, the less his or her overt competence becomes. A wide gap between the person's overt and covert competence means that the person will function on a level much lower than he is capable of (Svensson, 1984). He or she will consequently receive more care than needed and be 'forced' into dependency. This reaction to poorly adapted environments is true for those that under-utilize as well as over-strain the person's abilities. Over-stimulation as well as under-stimulation probably contributes to maladaptive behaviour. This idea has been put forward to explain the development of disruptive behaviour in severely demented people (Miller, 1977; Hallberg, 1990). Disruptive behaviour may be a reaction to badly-adapted environmental conditions (Haugen, 1985). The nursing home care of demented people was found to embody under-stimulation in the form of patients spending most of their time in a chair, often behind a safety tray. Nobody was within reach to involve them in meaningful activities (Hallberg *et al.*, 1990a). The care was also characterized by short, rapid, fragmentary nurse–patient interactions – the nurse frequently came and left the patient several times within the same care procedure (Hallberg *et al.*, 1990b).

This type of nurse–patient interaction is particularly damaging (iatrogenic) for people suffering from profound difficulties in perceptualizing and interpreting situations. Thus the care of these patients seemed to under-stimulate as well as over-stimulate them. The care may have contributed to the development of the vocally disruptive behaviour. This interpretation was further supported in a study exploring the relationship between vocally disruptive behaviour after lunch and the nurse–patient verbal interaction. The occurrence of vocally disruptive behaviour showed a significant relationship to nurses' interacting in a harsh tone of voice (Edberg *et al.*, 1995). Nurse–patient cooperation has also been found to become less a matter of exercising power over the patient, and more the patient becoming increasingly active during a 1-year intervention with clinical supervision and the implementation of planned individual care (Hallberg *et al.*, 1995; Edberg *et al.*, 1996).

Thus, if the needs assessment focuses only on the care recipients and does not take contextual factors into consideration, a dangerous reduction is made regarding the care recipient. To pinpoint poorly adapted environmental conditions, they need to be included when the care needs of a person are assessed.

A multidimensional approach to needs assessment

Based on the research findings, and other theories, a model was developed for needs assessment in cases where the elderly person suffered from cognitive impairment/reduced communicative abilities. The model was based on the idea that care should cover the needs that a person without communication difficulties would have; prevailing environmental conditions would be assessed. Three main aspects of an elderly person's life were selected for the different perspectives of assembling information (Figure 6.1):

- The person in an historical perspective
- The person in the present
- The person's closest environmental context in time as well as in space.

The person in an historical perspective

One dominant perspective will have shaped the present situation. Therefore it is necessary to gain an understanding of the *person's life story* and personality as it functioned during the healthy part of his or her life.

The person's life story includes the physical as well as the

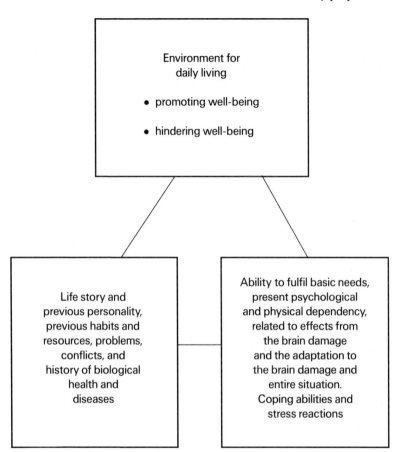

Figure 6.1 Various aspects of a cognitively impaired person's life that need to be covered in the process of needs assessments

psychosocial life story. During their lifetime a person lives through many events of a physical nature (e.g. traumatic incidents that have resulted in lasting dysfunctions), such as a damaged knee from playing football or a damaged back from working hard in a household, perhaps accompanied by chronic pain. For a lifetime the person has had habits of a physical nature (e.g. some people have kept and developed good physical condition and always liked to be 'on the run'; others have liked to live a lazy life, resting or laying down in the sun or reading rather than running around). The person may have had diseases and adjusted to these in various ways. Some diseases progress slowly throughout life and may give rise to later symptoms. Care recipients may be hindered in telling about these symptoms because of their communication difficulties.

Case example
An elderly woman could not express herself in verbal communication and seemingly had severe problems in understanding others. She shouted loudly and heart-rendingly, especially during the morning care and when she was spoon fed. She often refused to eat. It was noted in the medical record that she had a malignant cancer in her womb. It had been discovered during a regular cytological test but had produced no symptoms. It had been decided not to treat the cancer due to her dementia. Shortly after this the woman died and the autopsy revealed that she had metastases all over her body. While alive the woman had had no pain killers; seemingly pain from the progressing cancer was the explanation for her shouting.

Thus there is a need to plot the person's physical life story from the perspective of habits, likes and dislikes and from the perspective of reduced functions or diseases that the person has been living with and adjusted to over most of their life time. Understanding the person's physical life story means gathering data on the objective facts of their previous physical health as well as of their coping and adjustment to their physical health and reduction of their abilities.

The other part of their life story that needs to be assessed is the *psychosocial life history*. This part includes assessing the person's *previous personality* as well as the events and habits of a *psychosocial nature*. These other factors have taken place or developed during their life time and seemingly have had a formative impact on their life style (Hagberg, 1989). The person may for instance have had a long-standing habit of getting close to other people, telling all about themselves, trusting other people's positive attitude. They may have had special relations with people of the opposite sex. For instance the woman who has never had close relationships with a man may feel threatened when a male nurse enters the room and starts to take off her nightgown.

People have different ways of reacting in threatening or demanding situations, for instance, crises or situations that involve personal threats. Some people react by telling everybody about their problems. Others react with anger and explain the situation by blaming others. Other people blame themselves or turn inwards, telling nothing about their agony or sorrow. For instance, it was found in an explorative study that previously being introvert, keeping emotions inside and being anxious was significantly related to the development of vocally disruptive behaviour during the course of dementia (Holst *et al.*, 1997). Care recipients who developed such behaviour (apart from influence from the present environmental conditions) may have had an anxious and introverted previous personality that they were able to adapt to prior to the onset of dementia. When the disease progressed, it also destroyed their mode of adaptation and more of the anxiety came out into the open. The person may also have been through situations that have formed their life and reactions to various events.

Case example
An elderly demented woman always looked terrified when the staff came to help her out of bed, want to give her a shower or to help her to the toilet. She holds on to their trousers or doors, and often puts her hands over her head as if to protect it from blows. In her life history assessment, made in collaboration with her best friend, it was revealed that she had been battered throughout her married life.

It may well be that recent traumatic events are also stored as an emotional memory that causes reactions in similar situations. This has not been the focus of research. In regular clinical supervision sessions, however, caregivers repeatedly described situations which indicated that the care recipient (in spite of severe memory deficits) remembered recent traumatic events, and reacted to various situations similar to the actual traumatic situation. For instance, the person who had been through an episode of traumatic physical treatment (and reacted with severe panic during it) also reacted whenever the staff approached the same body area on which the treatment had focused, as if it were that particular situation acted out again. Thus she panicked whenever the staff came close to that area unless they approached her with exaggerated care.

These findings require systematic investigation. Even though this is lacking, assessing important life events should also cover recent events and reactions. This may help caregivers to understand strong emotional reactions and avoid arousing catastrophic reactions (Goldstein, 1952). Thus, understanding a person in his or her present life situation requires assessing their life history, significant psychosocial life events, traumatic life events (including events that have taken place recently). It should also include an assessment of the person's physical health history, as well as any disease that may progress (or in other respects have an impact) on their current health and infirmities.

This kind of information can be gathered from the care recipient's next of kin, husband, wife, children, close friends and neighbours. It cannot be gathered all at once. The basic information can be collected in one or two planned interviews with the closest relatives. Apart from these planned interviews, to understand and interpret properly the care recipient, an ongoing discussion between professional carers and the next of kin is required. This permits continuous collection of the information needed. For instance, the caregiver can tell stories from everyday care and ask the families to reflect on them and give their interpretations and their reasons for a particular interpretation.

The person in the present

The other perspective for needs assessment is the person at present, i.e. the present psychosocial and physical functional ability as it has been influenced by the disease(s) and the adaptation to the disease(s). In the case of dementia this means assessing the brain damage as it has affected the person's functional ability (Carnevali and Thomas, 1993). For instance, localizations to the frontal lobe give rise more to 'personality' changes (Wallin et al., 1994). Dementia of the Alzheimer's type gives rise more to memory and orientation problems (Wallin et al., 1994). Symptoms in vascular dementia disease depend on the area of the vascular damage (Wallin et al., 1994). The diseases are at various stages when the care recipients' needs are to be assessed and the progress varies in pace and in localization. Thus there is no simple relationship between disease and decreased functional ability. Also, the state changes over time, and this calls for repeated assessment.

In the intervention study to increase the quality of care by means of systematic clinical supervision and supervised planning of individualized care, it was decided to focus on the following areas in the care plans: the patients' ability to handle rest and activity, mobility, personal hygiene and dressing, elimination and toilet routines, nutrition, social involvement and individual adaptive resources, personal temper and mood (Berg et al., 1994; Edberg et al., 1996). These areas formed the key words for the care plan and each patient was carefully assessed to find where there were abilities left, and how the reduced abilities within the particular domain were damaged. In the implementation of planned individualized care it was found to be difficult to hinder the staff from defining the patients' need on the basis of what they provided in terms of help and support. This coincides with the statement by McWalter *et al.* (1994) that there is a tendency to 'think in terms of services rather than needs' (p. 213).

In the case of elderly people other diseases emerge and progress. Thus there is the need to focus not only on the consequences of the main disease (e.g. dementia disease). Elderly people often suffer from several diseases (Österlind, 1993). If the person has communication problems s/he cannot easily tell caregivers about symptoms from other diseases. In the case of elderly demented people one may decide that some diseases should not be treated, for instance cancer. However, the disease may have symptoms that require palliative care and since the patient cannot describe the symptoms (e.g. 'I am in pain'), then staff have to be alert to the type of symptoms that accompany other conditions. Pain and the alleviation of pain may also be of importance because elderly people's bodies are affected by the hard work they did during their life time. This body pain may increase because the person is bedridden, or has to spend hours in a chair in the same position, and with restricted ability to change the body position.

The assessment of physical aspects mentioned above needs to be an amalgamation of various diseases and their effects on functional abilities. In order to amalgamate these aspects into each other, knowledge is needed about the disease as well as its impact on functional ability. There is, however, a need also to assess and integrate the person's adaptation to the disease (i.e. how the person copes with the disease and its effects), as well as how the person reacts to situations that involve stress (e.g. the demands of the situation exceed the person's abilities to deal with it).

The coping strategies are believed to be formed throughout life, meaning that the life history assessment provides information about earlier strategies (Hagberg, 1989). These earlier strategies, however, need to be confirmed by the descriptions of the person's present reactions to new and stressful events. As for demented people it is common to differentiate between primary and secondary symptoms. Primary symptoms are believed to be directly related to the brain damage, while the secondary symptoms are related to coping and adjusting to the effects of the disease. Among the coping strategies, in the case of early dementia, there are adaptation strategies such as avoiding stressful events or situations that the person no longer has the resources to deal with. For instance, this involves withdrawing from socializing with others, not keeping up former habits which exceed their current capacity. There are reactions of paranoia, for example, and reactions indicating a complete functional collapse resulting, for instance, in outbursts, aggressive actions or crying, e.g. catastrophic reactions.

Another perspective for assessing the effects of the disease is trying to extract the existential meaning and living situation that the person experiences at present. It has, for instance, been stated that some demented people suffer from deep feelings about homelessness which inform their actions (Zingmark *et al.*, 1993). The life situation of others may be marked by the fact that they have no situational understanding at all. This means the care situations are often seen and reacted to as if they were life-threatening (Hallberg, 1995). In other cases, the dementia disease means that people seem totally to lose orientation, implying that they need the constant presence of another person in order not to feel completely lost. These people are often experienced as extremely tiring since they constantly ask for reassurance about where they are, where to go, and what is going to happen next. They often forget that they asked the same question ten seconds ago and were given an answer. Their inner state seems to be dominated by an inner feeling of being 'cast out into the universe' (Hallberg, 1995). Others may act and react to the present as if the time span had shattered completely. They act as they did in their healthy life and people around them in their present situation replace the former important actors in the care recipient's life.

For instance, the other care recipients are treated as if they were the children of the care recipient, or employees that have played an important part in the person's previous life. This situation may cause safety risks or inconvenience for other care recipients as well as for the person. Thus there is also the need to explore the meaning of the disease and the adjustment to it, for the person in order to understand fully what the existential meaning of living is with that particular situation.

Thus, there is a need to assess the effects of the disease(s) and the adaptation to them from physical, psychosocial and existential perspectives, and to interpret and integrate that knowledge into the frame of everyday care. Information can be collected from one's own as well as from others' systematic and arbitrary observations, from medical investigations and records and neuropsychological tests. It is also necessary to set up test situations that are carefully monitored in order to discover the boundary between ability and reduced ability and to understand the specifics of the reduction of ability.

For instance this may include difficulties in perception (i.e. 'see, recognize and understanding of the meaning of a plate with food in front of me'). It may mean 'problems maintaining concentration and focusing on eating, especially when it is noisy and I hear a lot of conversations going on and I am not certain whether they pertain to me'. It may mean that 'I have difficulties in differentiating between my plate and that of the person nearest me, so that every now and then I take food from plates other than my own and others may get very angry with me'. It may mean that 'I have severe difficulties in chewing and swallowing the food due to damage similar to those from Parkinson's disease and that the risk of aspirating food hangs over me, especially in a noisy environment' (see Norberg and Athlin, 1987).

The person's environmental context

The third perspective for the needs assessment is evaluating the care recipient's context in terms of how well the environment is adapted to his or her needs. Environment can be assessed from various perspectives. Lawton (1980) presents five aspects of the environment: personal environment, group environment, suprapersonal environment, social environment and physical environment. Examples of some of these aspects are given below. All aspects are of relevance for severely demented people as they are victims of the conditions and have only limited resources for altering or withdrawing from badly adapted environmental conditions or for adapting themselves to those conditions. Environmental aspects can be assessed from what the care recipient needs in the way of support or qualities from the surroundings; it can also be assessed from the aspect of iatrogenic influences from the environmental factors.

The *personal environment* is made up of significant others, family as well as (for instance) primary formal caregiver. The qualities of their relationships as well as the availability of significant others, are aspects to be assessed which have an impact on the care recipient's daily living. There may (for instance) be nobody there, ever, to reassure the person about his or her existence. The importance for human existence of being confirmed in relationships in order to keep up a picture of oneself as an important other has been emphasized (Watzlavick *et al.*, 1967; Gustafsson and Pörn, 1994). In contrast to that idea, it has been found that care of the severely demented tends to isolate and under-stimulate the care recipients in terms of activities, as well as interactions with important others (Hallberg *et al.*, 1990a,b).

The *group environment* means the relationship between the subject and the entire group of actors in that environment (i.e. staff as well as fellow patients). In the case of caring for the elderly, the group environment may mean that there are conflicts between care recipients that badly affect their daily life. The overall climate may be of a harsh or of a friendly type affecting individuals. These aspects are influenced very much by the way a group of care recipients are put together and the attitudes and actions of the staff. Small homogeneous groups of people with staff support have been emphasized as the means of achieving the best possible group climate (Annerstedt, 1995).

The *physical environment* is of great importance for demented people as well as for other diseased elderly people. It has been stated that the physical environment needs to be characterized by stability and clarity in cues (Roberts and Algase, 1988). This applies not only to the physical aspects like furniture, beds, rooms, sounds and lights in the environment, it also applies to the caregivers' routines and ways of performing care procedures. It may mean that there is a tradition among caregivers of staying with a patient after waking them up – helping them to get out of bed, shower or have a bath and dress – until they are ready for breakfast, without letting anybody interrupt the performance of the procedure and without leaving the care recipient for any reason.

There may be the opposite way of performing care, coming and leaving, speaking with others not involved in the procedure or letting others interfere with the procedure (Hallberg *et al.*, 1990b, 1995). This is of great importance for the patient's well-being and actions and reactions in the situation and may be the reason for what others see as disruptive behaviour. Unfortunately, most research on disruptive behaviour together with dementia progress does not take environmental conditions into consideration (Cohen-Mansfield *et al.*, 1990). This shortcoming also goes for the assessment of such things as anxiety, aggressive actions and hostility.

The problems of having lived under environmental pressure may well go with people moving from one care context to another in order to be examined and treated. The care recipient suffering from progressive dementia and coming from their home or from some residential living or nursing home may have lived the last few months under severe environmental conditions (e.g. lying on a bed all day, with nobody knocking on their door since the ideology is not to override people's integrity). Nobody will involve them in activities and they may not dare to leave their bed or go outside their door since they are not certain of being able to find the way back. Assessing the person for dementia or for their needs on the basis of behaviour (without taking the environmental conditions into consideration) means environmental conditions may be assessed instead, rather than the care recipient's needs.

In conclusion, the needs assessment must also take into consideration the environmental conditions that are putting pressure on the care recipient. This assessment needs to be made reflecting various environmental conditions and related to the individual's needs and the iatrogenic effect that environment may have on that particular care recipient. This can be done, for instance, by assessing one day, or several, from noon to night, including the activities that take place, the quality of interactions, the care recipient's reactions and the physical and psychosocial surroundings.

Another approach may be to assess various situations that may be especially devastating for the care recipient. For instance the staff complained that the care recipients were extremely noisy during lunch hours. In order to understand this further, a sample of lunch hours were video-recorded and thereafter viewed and evaluated by the care staff and the researchers in collaboration. Then the sources of noise could be identified and steps taken. Predominantly noise was a result of the way the staff acted and this increased anxious behaviour and noise from the patients (e.g. the noise from the patients was interpreted as a reaction to the way the nurses acted in the situation).

Putting the pieces into an interpreted whole about needs to be met in care

The collecting of information from various perspectives needs to be interpreted in order to be able to state what the needs of a care recipient are, what needs it is possible to meet and how to meet those needs. Reliability and validity in needs assessment for individuals rest in the assessment being right for that individual, not that it is being performed in the same manner for all other care recipients. It is not a single event, at least in the care of the demented. It is a continuous process that needs reflective discussion over and over to make sure that the care provided is really adjusted to the needs of that individual person. Thus the care organization requires a system that sets the primary caregiver in the right direction in assessing the patient from the various perspectives (see Figure 6.1). It should help to keep in mind the various aspects that should to be covered within each perspective. The care organization needs a structure for continuous reflective discussions about how to interpret a care recipient's needs and how to meet those needs (Schön, 1983). Systematic clinical supervision, in combination with supervised planning of individualized care, proved to serve the staffs' job satisfaction and creativity as well as the quality of care and care recipients' well-being (Hallberg and Norberg, 1993; Berg *et al.*, 1994; Hallberg *et al.*, 1994, 1995; Edberg *et al.*, 1996).

It is worthwhile to aim for dynamic models for needs assessment in the elderly, especially with those who are confused or demented. Continuous interpretation of the information is required and interpretation of which needs can be met, and how to meet them.

References

Annerstedt, L. (1995) *On Group-living Care for the Demented Elderly. Experiences from the Malmö Model.* Thesis. Department of Community Health Sciences, Malmö and Department of Geriatric Psychiatry, University of Lund, Sweden.

Berg, A., Welander Hansson, U., Hallberg, I. R. (1994) Nurses' creativity, tedium and burnout during 1 year of clinical supervision and implementation of individually planned care: comparisons between a ward for severely demented patients and a similar control ward. *Journal of Advanced Nursing,* 20, 742–749.

Carnevali, D., Thomas, M. D. (1993) *Diagnostic Reasoning Treatment Decision Making in Nursing.* Philadelphia: J.B. Lippincott Company.

Cohen-Mansfield, J., Werner, P., Marx, M. S. (1990) Screaming in nursing home residents. *Journal of the American Geriatric Society,* 38, 785–792.

Edberg, A-K., Nordmark Sandgren, Å., Hallberg, I. R. (1995) Initiating and terminating verbal interaction between nurses and severely demented patients regarded as vocally disruptive. *Journal of Psychiatric Nursing,* 2, 159–167.

Edberg, A-K., Hallberg, I. R., Gustafson, L. (1996) Effects of clinical supervision on nurse–patient cooperation quality. A controlled study in dementia care. *Clinical Nursing Research,* 5, 127–149.

Ehnfors, M., Thorell-Ekstrand, I., Ehrenberg, A. (1991) Towards basic nursing information in patient records. *Vård i Norden,* 21, 12–31.

Goldstein, K. (1952) The effect of brain damage on the personality. *Psychiatry,* 15, 245–260.

Gustafsson, B., Pörn, I. (1994) A motivational approach to confirmation: an interpretation of dysphagic patients' experiences. *Theoretical Medicine*, **15**, 353–369.

Hagberg, B. (1989) *The Individual Life History as a Formative Experience to Ageing*. Lund, Sweden: Gerontology Research Centre.

Hallberg, I. R. (1990) *Vocally Disruptive Behaviour in Severely Demented Patients in Relation to Institutional Care Provided*. Thesis. Umeå University Medical Dissertations. New series no. 261. Umeå, Sweden.

Hallberg, I. R. (1995) *Systematic Clinical Supervision and Individualized Nursing Care; the Effects on the Staff's Well-being, on the Care and on the Patients*. Stockholm: Liber Läromedel.

Hallberg, I. R., Norberg, A. (1993) Strain among nurses and their emotional reactions during one year of systematic clinical supervision combined with the implementation of individualized care in dementia care. Comparison between an experimental ward and a control ward. *Journal of Advanced Nursing*, **18**, 1860–1875.

Hallberg, I. R., Norberg, A., Eriksson, S. (1990a) A comparison between the care of vocally disruptive patients and that of other residents at psychogeriatric wards. *Journal of Advanced Nursing*, **15**, 410–416.

Hallberg, I. R., Luker, K. A., Norberg, A., Johnsson, K., Eriksson, S. (1990b) Staff interaction with vocally disruptive demented patients compared with demented controls. *Aging*, **2**, 163–171.

Hallberg, I. R., Holst, G., Nordmark, Å., Edberg, A-K. (1995) Cooperation during morning care between nurses and severely demented institutionalized patients. *Clinical Nursing Research*, **4**, 78–104.

Hallberg, I. R., Welander Hansson, U. W., Axelsson, K. (1994) Satisfaction with care and work during a year of clinical supervision and individualized care. *Journal of Nursing Management*, **1**, 297–307.

Haugen, P. K. (1985) Behaviour of patients with dementia. *Danish Medical Bulletin*, **32**, suppl. 1, 62–65.

Heston, L. L., Garrard, J., Makris, L., Kane, R. L., Cooper, S., Dunham, T. et al. (1992) Inadequate treatment of depressed nursing home elderly. *Journal of the American Geriatric Society*, **40**, 1117–1122.

Holst, G., Hallberg, I. R., Gustafson, L. (1997) The relationship of vocally disruptive and previous personality in severely demented institutionalized patients. *Archives of Psychiatric Nursing*, **11**, 147–154.

Lawton, M. P. (1980) *Environment of Aging*. Monterey, California: Brooks/Cole Publishing Company.

Maslow, A. H. (1954) *Motivation and Personality*. New York: Harper.

McLean, S. (1987a) Assessing dementia. Part I: Difficulties, definition and differential diagnosis. *Australian and New Zealand Journal of Psychiatry*, **21**, 142–174.

McLean, S. (1987b) Review. Assessing dementia. Part II: Clinical, functional, neuropsychological and social issues. *Australian and New Zealand Journal of Psychiatry*, **21**, 284–304.

McWalter, G., Toner, H., Corser, A., Eastwood, J., Marshall, M., Turvey T. (1994) Needs and needs assessment: their components and definitions with reference to dementia. *Health and Social Care*, **2**, 213–219.

Miller, E. (1977). The management of dementia: a review of some possibilities. *British Journal of Social and Clinical Psychology*, **16**, 77–83.

Norberg, A., Athlin, E. (1987) The interaction between the Parkinsonian patient and his caregiver during feeding: a theoretical model. *Journal of Advanced Nursing*, **12**, 545–550.

Österlind, P. O. (1993) *Medical and Social Conditions in the Elderly Gender and Age Differences. The Umeå Longitudinal Study.* Thesis. Department of Geriatric Medicine, University of Umeå, Umeå, Sweden.

Roberts, B. L., Algase, D. L. (1988) Victims of Alzheimer's disease and the environment. *Nursing Clinics of North America*, **23**, 83–94.

Schön, A. (1983) *The Reflective Practitioner. How Professionals Think in Action.* London: Maurice Temple Smith Ltd.

Svensson, T. (1984) *Aging and Environment. Institutional Aspects.* Thesis. Linköping Studies in Education Dissertations no. 21, Linköping University, Sweden.

The National Board of Health and Welfare (1993) *Health Care and Social Service in Seven European Countries* no. 6, Stockholm, Sweden.

Wallin, A., Brun, A., Gustafson, L. (1994) Swedish consensus on dementia diseases. *Acta Neurologica Scandinavica*, **90**, 8–31.

Watzlavick, P., Bavelas, J. B., Jackson, D. D. (1967) *Pragmatics of Human Communication. A Study of Interactional Patterns, Pathologies and Paradoxes.* New York: Norton & Company Inc.

Zingmark, K., Norberg, A., Sandman, P. O. (1993) Experience of at-homeness and homesickness in patients with Alzheimer's disease. *American Journal of Alzheimer Care and Related Disease Research*, **8**, 10–16.

Chapter 7

The antinomies of choice in community care

Kirsten Stalker

Introduction

The notion of choice is a recurring theme in community care. The White Paper, 'Caring for People: Community Care in the Next Decade and Beyond' (Secretaries of State for Health, Social Security, Wales and Scotland, 1989), which in Britain preceded the National Health Service and Community Care Act (1990), asserts that 'promoting choice and independence underlies all the Government's proposals' (1.8). The focus on choice is echoed, and fleshed out in policy and practice terms, in the various documents of guidance accompanying the legislation, and in community care plans across the country. The need to promote choice – or the right to exercise it – has been championed by a broad spectrum of political, professional and 'user' opinion. But what exactly is meant by choice? What conceptual or theoretical assumptions underpin it and what do these indicate about current policy initiatives? These are large questions which cannot be fully answered in this short chapter. An attempt will be made, however, to explore 'choice' at both conceptual and policy levels, looking at the different traditions which inform current use of the word. Some implications will be drawn out about the nature of 'choice' within the context of community care.

At first glance, perhaps, 'choice' may seem a relatively simple term, denoting the act of choosing between two or more alternatives. The Oxford Advanced Learners' Dictionary cites eight different meanings, but the sense and implications of the word will also vary in relation to the theoretical context in which it is being used at any time. Choice is currently a fashionable term. Generally perceived as 'a good thing', few would argue against it in principle. In this sense, it is similar to the word 'community' which, as Williams (1989) points out: 'is unusual among the terms of political vocabulary as the one term which has never been used in a negative sense. People never, from any political persuasion, want to say they are 'against community or against the community'.

Williams cautions that any word which attracts almost universal approval should also arouse some suspicion. The ability of one concept to be 'all things to all people' is a curious phenomenon. One way to approach this question is to think of a concept dialectically, that is, as more than just an abstract notion; it is also an intellectual representation of something which has a tangible or real-life form. The German philosopher Adorno referred to an 'unfulfilled' concept to indicate one which is not sufficiently coherent in the abstract to be fully 'realized' in practice, thus creating antinomies, or contradictions, in real life (Adorno, 1973). Within this framework, the nature of 'choice' in community care will be explored.

Choice and empowerment

Central to community care is the notion of user empowerment and it is in this language that the concept of choice is often, although not always, couched. The clearest 'official' articulation of choice in this sense is contained in the following statement in 'Care Management and Assessment: Summary of Practice Guidance':

> The rationale for this re-organisation is the empowerment of users and carers. Instead of users being subordinate to the wishes of service-providers, the roles will be progressively adjusted (SSI/SWSG, 1991a, p. 7).

In 'Caring for People' it is stated that the reforms offer 'better quality and choice' than other forms of support, and that they are intended to give people greater individual say in how they live their lives. Assessment should take account of the individual's wishes, and those of carers (raising the question, incidentally, of whose choice is to be met, where differences arise, and how conflicting choices are to be reconciled). Individuals and carers are to be offered flexible services which enable them to make choices (3.2.6). Care managers are expected actively to involve individuals in the assessment process:

Wherever possible, users should be offered a genuine choice of service options, appropriate to their ethnic and cultural background. This enables them to feel that they have some control over what is happening to them and reinforces their sense of independence (SSI/SWSG, 1991b, p. 63).

The promotion of choice in the sense of gaining empowerment and independence is not unique to community care. It is given prominence in the ethos of normalization, for example, as one of O'Brien's (1987) 'Five Accomplishments' for service delivery. Similarly, the Wagner Report (1988) discusses choice in the sense of the empowerment, or disempowerment, of elderly people in residential care. The report's conclusions are echoed in the White Paper's statements that admission to residential or nursing care should always be seen as a 'positive choice'.

Croft and Beresford (1993) distinguish between what they see as two different types of user involvement in service development, the 'democratic' and the 'consumerist'. The democratic approach:

> aims to empower people by giving them a voice in organizations and services. Power and changes in the distribution of power are central to this model. It is concerned with people as citizens. A democratic approach is most clearly associated with schemes to increase people's direct involvement in decision-making (p. 21).

Thus, the authors identify an attempt to empower people in the 'democratic' model but not in the 'consumerist' model (as will be discussed later). Empowerment is, however, becoming an over-worked word, since it is increasingly used to signify a range of differing levels of user involvement and not necessarily a real 'taking on' or 'over' of power by the service user from the service provider. This is illustrated, at policy and practice level, in a continuum of involvement in service planning and delivery, comprising four levels, developed by Fiedler and Twitchin (1992). These range from 'information-giving' and 'consultation' to 'partnership' and 'delegated control'. The last of these, arguably the closest to empowerment, involves service users given the funding, and authority, to plan, implement and manage services. Such developments are now under way in relation to coalitions of disabled people in some parts of the country. An example at individual level is a person acting as his or her own care manager, or employing their own personal assistants through Independent Living Fund monies.

Self-determination

Running throughout the examples and extracts quoted above is the common thread of choice. It is being used in relation to people gaining greater control over their lives, beginning to set their own agendas, rather than responding to those laid down by professionals. This appears to be choice in the tradition of self-determination. That is not to say that self-determination will be the outcome of present policies, nor that such is the government's intention. It has also been forcibly argued that the principles underlying 'community care' are not compatible with those of 'Independent Living', and that the notion of professionally-assessed needs is at odds with disabled peoples' demands for rights and entitlements (Oliver, 1990; Morris, 1994). Much of the language of choice as presented and reproduced within community care uses the vocabulary of self-determination and appears to draw from that tradition.

The idea of self-determination has received considerable attention at different stages in the development of Western philosophy, both in relation to the individual, as in the work of Kant and Fichte, and in relation to society as a whole, as developed by Hegel and, later, by Marx. It is characterized in part by a belief in people as autonomous beings, capable of exercising free and rational choice. There is also a conviction that human beings have the right to do so. Kant condemned the 'despotism of paternalism' which manipulates others according to its own idea of what is good for them, rather than encouraging people to formulate their own wishes, choices and decisions. The goals of self-determination can be achieved through decision-making structures in which all citizens can participate. According to this construction, the exercise of choice is seen as a significant step along the road to self-determination.

The value of self-determination has a long history within social work theory and practice, where it has attracted both champions and detractors. It has emerged in a number of guises, but for many years was seen primarily in relation to individual growth and self-development, representing: 'the exercise in very ordinary, and perhaps even foolish ways, of the powers of deliberation and choice the client already possesses' (McDermott, 1975, p. 7).

More recently, it has found expression in the activities of campaigning or lobbying groups, particularly in community development work, where people organize collectively and are not cast in the role of 'clients'. Those aspects of community care in which choice is associated with ideas of empowerment are clearly derived from the same tradition.

Choice and the mixed economy of care

However, the concept of choice is linked to another set of ideas within the 'new community care' which differ in nature and implication. The unifying principle is the mixed economy of welfare which the reforms are intended to promote and which are expected to widen the range of choices for 'consumers'. Since the early 1980s, local government has been undergoing radical changes as a result of successive pieces of legislation intended to stem its role as a public sector provider, for example, in the fields of housing and education (Caulfield and Schultz, 1989). Similarly, the development of a market in welfare, matched by the change in role for social work departments from providers to enablers, is a major policy objective of community care.

'Caring for People' sets out the government's expectation that local authorities will make use of a range of providers: 'in so far as this represents a cost-effective choice' and take 'all reasonable steps to secure diversity of provision' (3.4.1). Individuals should not be denied the opportunity to enter residential care within the independent sector, a policy which has become mandatory through the Direction on Choice of Accommodation (Scottish Office, 1993) under which authorities must place individuals in their 'preferred accommodation', provided it is suitable, available and affordable. It is predicted that stimulating the development of non-statutory services will result in 'a wider range of choice' for 'the consumer' (Caring for People, 3.4.3). Certain areas of provision are identified in which people have less choice than others, due to the slow pace of development in the independent sector. A number of strategies are identified whereby authorities can promote a mixed economy of care, including wider use of service specification and tendering. The Manager's Guide to Care Management and Assessment (SSI/SWSG, 1991c) spells out the structural arrangements required: the establishment of devolved budgeting and the separation of provider and purchaser wings of the department. A role is envisaged for staff to develop entrepreneurial skills.

These arrangements correspond to the 'consumerist' model of user involvement described by Croft and Beresford (1993) as:

The consumerist approach is service centred. The term consumer describes people in terms of their relationship with a product or service. This approach places an emphasis on 'exit', that is to say, people's ability to turn to another service if they are dissatisfied. Power remains with services and their providers. People can feed in their ideas and experience but agencies still make decisions (p. 21).

The market

In the extracts quoted above, choice is not presented in terms of self-determination but is used in a different sense (and drawing from a different line of thought) – 'the market'. This is made explicit in the guidance in references to establishing 'a market situation in which assessing staff are able to choose between provision in the statutory and independent sectors', thus also 'progressively expanding the choices available to users' and allowing in-house services 'to compete in the open market' (p. 36). Le Grand (1990) has suggested that 'quasi-market' is a more accurate formulation, since it differs from conventional markets in certain aspects of supply and demand.

'The market' has long been a central tenet of political economy, from the classical economist Adam Smith to neo-liberal thinkers such as Hayek and Friedman. At first sight, it may not appear to be a same order concept as 'self-determination'. Fredric Jameson (1991), however, is one writer who argues that the function of the market is primarily ideological rather than material. While it shares some of the vocabulary of self-determination (including freedom of choice) it differs from the other in its underlying assumptions. Here, public good is seen as arising from private gain. The market is believed to be the best means of ensuring economic efficiency, social justice and political freedom. Great emphasis is placed on individual responsibility, in the sense of being able to meet one's own needs, as opposed to collective or social responsibility: 'It is not from the benevolence of the butcher, the brewer or the baker that we expect our dinner, but from their regard to their own interest' (Smith, 1954).

Collective decision-making or, in policy terms, public planning, is considered inefficient, since not only does it restrict economic growth, but it also denies individual citizens their freedom of choice. Left to their own devices, competitive markets will ensure the most effective use of resources, thus creating a range of options. Individuals must have the right to assert their own preferences and act on their choices.

A divided unity

Thus far, it has been argued that 'choice' is used in community care policy 'talk' in two different ways. First it is used as part of promoting individual empowerment; second it is used within the context of a mixed economy of welfare. In the former sense, choice can be linked to the concept of self-determination, in the latter, to that of the market. Thus, two different conceptualizations are contained or perhaps concealed within the one word. Such a juxtaposition blurs differing ethos in current policy initiatives, yet it succeeds in winning unanimous approval for the concept. This does not resolve the central problem, however: 'choice' is an unfulfilled concept. It cannot represent a coherent whole and therefore will create contradictions in real life. It contains two ideas or arguments, one of which is likely to prevent the other from being fully realized at policy level. Again, there is a similarity with the word 'community', as analysed by Williams (1981), in relation to both the nature of the complexity of the concept and also, to some extent, its substantive content:

> The complexity of 'community' relates to the difficult interaction between the tendencies originally distinguished in the historical development: on the one hand, the sense of direct common concern; on the other hand, the materialization of various forms of common organization, which may or may not adequately express this (p. 76).

What are the difficulties in implementation which arise from the dual nature of choice in community care? Several can be identified. There are elements inherent in the market which, while perhaps increasing choice for a few, reduce it for many others. The arguments were clearly set out nearly 30 years ago by Titmuss (1968), but still hold good. Private markets are likely to exacerbate the problem of stigma and discrimination in welfare provision, with public services tending to be of a lower quality than those in the private sector, resulting in less freedom of choice. Again, because private markets depend on ability to pay, rather than criteria of need, Titmuss argues, they have the effect of further limiting choice in the public sector.

Further, because health and social services are significantly different in kind from other 'personal consumption goods' (particularly because of their uncertain and unpredictable nature) the scope for informed choice is far smaller. Finally, Titmuss contests the view that economic growth can adequately address poverty: redistributive social policies are also required.

Not only is the 'market' construction of choice limited in itself, it can also be expected to have certain detrimental effects, for example, in relation to equity, residualization and territorial justice. These factors are likely to undermine the extent to which choice, as a step along the road to self-determination, can really be offered within community care. Challis and Henwood (1994) predict that the degree to which social services departments will be able to influence the market will be extremely variable: 'depending on local conditions of supply and demand and the ideological stances adopted towards the independent sector... There will, in short, be inequity in the amount of choice available to people who need care' (p. 1498).

The harmful effects of charging policies which have accompanied the introduction of the market are already being seen (House of Commons Health Committee, 1993; Stalker *et al.*, 1994).

There are two possible outcomes to the antinomies of choice in community care. The first (which within the present analysis would be seen as an unhappy compromise) is a widespread establishment and acceptance of the market as the only framework in which choice is available. Furthermore, this construction of choice may be increasingly perceived not only as unproblematic conceptually, but as desirable in practice. Thus, while the individual is accorded the status of 'consumer' and allocated certain 'rights', such as the right to a quality service or the right to complain, her power to make real choices remains circumscribed by structures and forces largely beyond her control.

There is another possible outcome, however, to the divided unity of choice. It may be that service users, along with other groups and individuals, will find a way to reclaim the language and values of self-determination which the market has sought to appropriate. The disability 'movement' has demonstrated how much can be achieved by a relatively small number of people willing and able to demand the right to exercise choice and control over their lives. Other user groups and networks are gradually growing in strength and numbers. There are potential parallels with the experience of the women's movement.

Some people will choose not to become involved; others, for a variety of reasons, are unable to. Whether either of these (or other) outcomes will ensue, and the extent to which compromise or conflict will occur, is an interesting question for future theoretical and empirical research in community care.

Acknowledgements

I am grateful to Bill Munro and colleagues in the Department of Applied Social Science at Stirling University for their comments on this chapter.

References

Adorno, T. (1973) *Negative Dialectics*. London: Routledge.

Caulfield, I., Schultz, J. (1989) *Planning for Change: Strategic Planning in Local Government*, Harlow: Longman.

Challis, L., Henwood, M. (1994) Equity in community care. *British Medical Journal*, **308**, 1496–1499.

Croft, S., Beresford, P. (1993) *Getting Involved: a Practical Manual*, London: Open Services Project.

Fiedler, B., Twitchin, D. (1992) Achieving user participation. *Living Options in Practice Project, Paper no. 3.*

House of Commons Health Committee (1993) *Sixth Report Community Care – The Way Forward*, 1. London: HMSO.

Jameson, F. (1991) *Postmodernism or the Cultural Logic of Late Capitalism*. London: Verso.

Le Grand, J. (1990) *Quasi-markets and Social Policy, DQM No. 1*. Bristol: SAUS Publications, School for Advanced Urban Studies, University of Bristol.

McDermott, F. E. (1975) *Self-determination in Social Work*. London: Routledge and Kegan Paul.

Morris, J. (1994) *Independent Lives, Community Care and Disabled People*. London: Macmillan.

O'Brien, J. (1987) A guide to life style planning. In *A Comprehensive Guide to the Activities Catalogue: An Alternative Curriculum for Youth and Adults with Severe Disabilities* (B. Wilcox and G. T. Bellamy, eds). Baltimore: Paul H. Brookes.

Oliver, M. (1990) *The Politics of Disablement*. London: Macmillan.

Scottish Office (1993) Social Work (Scotland) Act 1968 (Choice of Accommodation) Directions 1993, Scottish Office Social Work Services Group, Circular no. SW05/1993, Edinburgh.

Secretaries of State for Health, Social Security, Wales and Scotland (1989) *Caring for People: Community Care in the Next Decade and Beyond*. London: HMSO.

Smith, A. (1954) *Wealth of Nations*. London: Dent Dutton.

SSI/SWSG (Social Services Inspectorate/Social Work Services Group) (1991a) *Care Management and Assessment: Summary of Practice Guidance*. London: HMSO.

SSI/SWSG (Social Services Inspectorate/Social Work Services Group) (1991b) *Care Management and Assessment: Practitioners' Guide*. London: HMSO.

SSI/SWSG (Social Services Inspectorate/Social Work Services Group) (1991c)

Care Management and Assessment: Managers' Guide. London: HMSO.

Stalker, K., Taylor, J., Petch, A. (1994) *Implementing Community Care in Scotland: Early Snapshots*. University of Stirling, Social Work Research Centre.

The Wagner Report (1988) *Residential Care. a Positive Choice*. London: HMSO.

Titmuss, R. (1968) Commitment to Welfare. London: Unwin.

Williams, R. (1981) *Keywords: a Vocabulary of Culture and Society*. London: Fontana (first published 1976).

Williams, R. (1989) *Resources of Hope*. London: Verso.

Chapter 8

Feminist perspectives on community care in Australia

Melanie Edwards

Introduction

In gender neutral language, neutrality has masked the engendered experiences which the word denotes. 'Community care', an expression which implies care by the community, disguises the fact that it is generally women who do the caring (Pascall, 1986). The term community care, rather than meaning care by the community, means care in the community (Mowbray and Bryson, 1984). Community care in Australia has been consistent with de-institutionalization in the UK and the USA, pushed by the former Labor government's pledge to privatization.

Privatization

In Australia, privatization at a community level has involved the transference of functions to the private sector in four ways (Moore, 1990):

1 contracting out services
2 public service abrogation
3 return of public responsibilities to individuals and their families
4 the use of charitable non-government organizations and volunteers.

One effect of this kind of privatization is the reliance on lowly paid or volunteer workers. As women are over-represented in these areas, they suffer disproportionately from any kind of privatization (Moore, 1990). Privatization can be seen as an economic decision, which forces care into the community when it becomes less viable for the government to support those who are institutionalized. As care is removed, and less money is provided for social services, clients and care givers suffer from the effects of economic rationalism.

Feminist theory

Feminism, feminist theory and its proponents, are attempts to 'describe women's oppression, to explain its causes and to prescribe strategies for women's liberation' (Tong, 1989, p. 1). Feminists have provided critiques of patriarchy and why it occurs. Feminist scholarship has been broken into branches according to differing conceptual frameworks. Walby (1990) makes the divisions between liberal feminism, Marxist feminism, radical feminism and the dual theorists. These branches are the most commonly referred to in economic discussion, due to the primacy of economic analysis in their agenda. Other contemporary feminist analysis, such as psychoanalytic feminism (e.g. Chodorow, 1978), French feminism/postmodern feminism (e.g. Iragaray, 1985) and cultural feminism (e.g. Dolan, 1991), have been preoccupied with the formations of subjectivity, and are not relevant to economic discussion (Beechy, 1987).

Liberal feminism

The two main assumptions of liberal feminism are: that in the public sphere women should be accepted on equal terms with men and the concept of an individual citizen occurs *within* the division between the spheres; the division of the spheres is a societal not ideological one (Tapper, 1986; Eisenstein, 1986). The concept of work within the analyses of liberal feminism is based on an individualistic, democratic framework whereby citizens perform paid work in the public sphere (Tapper, 1986; Tong, 1989). This concept of work does not require reformation for women's liberation, but rather women's equality stems from equal representation in the public sphere, as reforms are made within the status quo, women would be able to 'throw off' their conditioned sex roles and liberate themselves (Tapper, 1986; Tong, 1989). The term 'women's work' has been merely a descriptive term describing the work that women do, just as 'men's work' is separated from 'work', as the work of the citizen (Eisenstein, 1984). Recently this conceptualization of the societal division of the spheres has been changing, with an increase of literature about liberal feminism, housework and women's caring duties. It has been suggested that women will never gain equality in the public sphere while household responsibilities (including caring responsibilities) are not seen as the norm for men (Townsend, 1995). The concept of work formulated by liberal feminism takes the standard definition of work as paid in the public sphere and has started to incorporate women's unpaid labour.

Radical feminism

Radical feminism does not make an analysis of work central to its project but rather focuses on the controlling mechanisms of violence and sexuality (Walby, 1990). When work is incorporated into the theoretical framework it is critiqued in the same way as other phallocentric concepts; the reconceptualization of work to include women's experience is central to the concept of work. Consistent with the slogan, 'personal is political', work as only paid and outside the home has been critiqued as patriarchal (Solanas, 1971). Unpaid domestic work (including women's biological/reproductive/caring work) has been subordinated to support the system of paid work, which was created by men for their own benefit (Novarra, 1980).

Marxist feminism

Marxist feminism differs from a radical or liberal analysis as it proposes that gender inequalities stem from oppression under a capitalist system (Tong, 1989; Walby, 1990). The argument, based on Marx's writings, suggests that women of different classes suffer differently under capitalism (Tong, 1989), and takes an *historical materialist* approach to the study of labour and labour relations (Barrett, 1980; Tong, 1989). Marxist feminism stresses the importance of ideology in the formation of women's oppression (from Marx, 1972), although the material and the ideological cannot always be clearly separated (Barrett, 1980). Marxist feminism, like liberal feminism, is preoccupied with women's role in the public sphere and neglects the role which women are relegated to in the private sphere.

Dual systems theory

Dual systems theory is the theory that in society women suffer the effects of both capitalism and patriarchy; dual systems is the fusion of radical and Marxist feminist theories (Hartmann, 1981; Young, 1981; Walby, 1990; Delphy and Leonard, 1992). These theories vary as to the ways in which Capitalism and Patriarchy are combined, as either interrelated and analytically distinct (Hartmann, 1981; Walby, 1990) or as amalgamated into one form (Eisenstein, 1986). The main preoccupation of the dual theoretic approaches is the exploitation of women in the private sphere and how this has repercussions on their definition in the public sphere. The family is seen as the main site of oppression (Delphy and Leonard, 1992) and Patriarchal/Capitalistic oppression can be seen to affect women's position in the public sphere both through their subordination to the private sphere and their relegation to the most degraded areas of the public sphere (Hartmann, 1981), and the engenderization of women's work. The concept of work as only paid and undertaken in the public sphere is believed to contribute to the power structures which oppress women, so the concept of work is extended to include both paid and unpaid work, both inside and outside the public sphere and both productive and reproductive (Walby, 1990; Delphy and Leonard, 1992).

Economic rationalism as a masculinist discourse

The investigation of the divisions seen in western society as natural is common to all analysis, and demonstrates the divisions in western societies. Masculine traits are set aside from feminine traits, and the latter are constructed as natural or biological. Hence, the proposition of community care, based on economic rationalism, can be thought of as masculinist. Economics (the public sphere of masculine activity) and rationalism (a traditionally masculine trait) are combined to legitimize and perpetuate stereotypes of caring as a feminine trait, and thus women as caregivers. This ideological base acts as a form of domination over the carers, who are exploited for their unpaid labour within a capitalistic framework. This reliance on community care (due to economic decisions and government policies) has been supported by backlash from the New Right, through its renewed emphasis on the community, the family as a nuclear unit and mother-care (Mowbray and Bryson, 1984; Baldock, 1988; Moore, 1990)

Ideological emphasis on the family

The economic rationalist approach has been increasingly justified through the renewed emphasis of the family as an ideological support (Mowbray and Bryson, 1984; Baldock, 1988; Moore, 1990). Privatization of community facilities has not been sold in Australia, as it has been in the USA (Baldock, 1988). Yet the primacy of the family has been advanced as a reason for de-institutionalization (Creed and Tomlinson, 1984), with maternal deprivation studies being used to emphasize a more 'humane' form of care (Mowbray and Bryson, 1984).

The legitimization of women's caring role as natural is contradictory to the goals of anti-discrimination policies (Mowbray and Bryson, 1984) as the ideology of women's natural ability to care emphasizes the public/private split and demonstrates the Australian government's lack of intervention outside the public sphere into the private sphere. The patriarchal ideology of women's caring role is naturalized and the legitimization in the community leads to:

1 hide the social nature of relationships
2 hide the variability of social facts
3 hide the exploitation and oppression associated with them (Delphy and Leonard, 1992).

The Australian experience of community care is consistent with experiences in the UK with women as the clients and the caregivers.

Women as caregivers

Women as caregivers in western societies

In western societies, caring work is prescribed to women in two ways (Mowbray and Bryson, 1984):

1 unpaid social reproduction (which involves caregiving within the household and extended family, and the work which women do within the private sphere such as housework and sexual/emotion labour)
2 voluntary welfare work (this involves voluntary community participation such as volunteer work and care outside the family unit).

Both these forms of caring work are performed in the private sphere. Neither are seen as work, due to their location (i.e. in the private sphere women's work is not seen as work). In Australian society women perform both of these types of caring work, while still participating in the public sphere.

Women as carers in Australian society – social reproduction

Women's participation in the labour force is not the same as men's participation. The labour force participation rate of women is 51.3% compared to men's 72.0% (ABS Australian Bureau of Statistics, 1993a). Women comprise 67.0% of persons not in the labour force. Sixty-nine per cent report household duties or child care as their main reason for non-participation (ABS, 1993a). Of the men not in the labour force, only 4.0% list household duties or child care as their main activity (ABS, 1993a).

From these statistics women are still the primary caregivers in Australian society. This has had the effect of keeping 275 500 women out of the labour force compared to only 7400 men (ABS, 1993a). As women are pushed out of the labour force (due to their caring duties and the lack of flexibility of working hours), they suffer from social, economic and emotional consequences due to this decreased labour market participation.

Social consequences of caring

As women continue to dominate the private sphere, cultural stereotypes will continue (Creed and Tomlinson, 1984). Regardless of the compensatory measures in social policy and education, stereotypes of the mother as the primary caregiver will influence children as they prepare for their chosen roles in society. The private/public dichotomy will be perpetuated, with the primacy given to the public over the private.

Economic consequences of caring

As caregivers spend more time out of the labour force their chances of gaining employment decrease (Moore, 1990); this increases the individual's dependency on a partner or pension. This dependency also increases in sickness or older-age. The dependency of the carer then falls on the shoulders of another person to perform as carer. This causes a cycle which perpetuates.

Emotional consequence of caring

Often, the onset of a caring role will leave the carer unprepared for the role. This situation can cause the 'hidden patient' (Schultz, 1990), where the carer is not recognized as troubled or physically ill. In Kinnear and Graycar's (1984) analysis of Australian ageing and family dependency, the carers in their study suffered deteriorations in their life style. They found:

- 79% had less time for leisure time activities
- 84% suffered a deterioration in work performance (where they were in paid employment)
- 56% suffered a deteriorating relationship with their spouse
- 60% were less able to relax and sleep at night
- 51% were apprehensive about growing older
- 90% had a rapidly deteriorating relationship with brothers and sisters (Kinnear and Graycar, 1984).

They suggested that there are two levels of support needed to assist with the caring:

1   services to support the family unit
2   services to support the principal carer.

These two strategies, while effective, do not seek to address the questions of why women are still the primary caregivers, or seek to redress the status quo. Another problem is: who will provide these services, who will be the workers? Women's relegation to the private sphere will only be strengthened by the use of lowly paid or volunteer (women) workers to provide care to families and primary caregivers (Moore, 1990).

Women's voluntary welfare labour

Results of statistical time studies have suggested that in the breakdown of a 24-hour period, women and men spend similar times in unpaid voluntary work and community participation (women, 24 minutes, men, 20 minutes) (ABS, 1992). Men's unpaid work is most often with able-bodied persons and associated travel, women's work tends to lie in a caring capacity helping adults or undertaking community work (such as volunteering in neighbourhood centres) (ABS, 1992). Men's unpaid labour tends to increase significantly over the weekend period (from 20 to 37 minutes per day); women's labour also increases, although not to the same extent (from 24 to 30 minutes per day). Results of these time studies are deceptive. Separate studies have shown that women constitute significantly more participants, while men tend to spend more time in unpaid labour (ABS, 1992). Men also constitute over two-thirds of all unpaid coaches, administrators and volunteers in recreational activities (ABS, 1993b).

These time studies statistics are consistent with Baldock's (1988) proposition that men's volunteer work tends to be more prestigious (e.g. sport and recreation) so that men's private sphere activities are more visible than women's and are generally not viewed as 'volunteer work'. Volunteer work is seen as a feminine trait (i.e. altruistic) and in western societies feminine traits are generally degraded (Mowbray and Bryson, 1984; Baldock, 1988).

Women as clients

Women as clients in Australian society

Women are not an homogeneous group; problems occur when this is assumed. Baldwin (1993) has outlined seven need areas which clients require when being relocated (or kept) in the community:

1 education
2 health
3 relationships
4 leisure
5 mobility
6 meaningful daytime activity
7 residence
   (some people also include)
8 spirituality.

Women are sometimes classified as a special needs group (i.e. having additional needs above and beyond those listed here). Women use fertility clinics and 'reproductive services', which are an adjunct of generic health services. Generic refers to the normative health behaviours based on male health. The usage of this language is problematic; it classes women into the minority, whose health services are viewed as extra.

Structural problems with services

One aspect of community involvement in the care of women is self-help classes, run in the neighbourhood houses and centres. These groups face structural problems which must be addressed so that women feel comfortable in the group and want to return. These problems include:

(a) problems with seeing women as one; sisterhood, stemming from the early writings of the women's liberation movement, rejects the idea of separating women on the basis of 'us' and 'them'. This way of thinking denies women's specific experiences, as not all women face the same oppression and class the same importance to varying experiences;

(b) the false equality trap; in community work, the volunteer or activist may fall into a trap whereby she 'strives to foster the myth of equality between herself and the rest of the group'. This position is 'potentially patronising, divisive and elitist' (Barker, 1986, p. 82);

(c) structural position of the group; as the leader of a group, attempts to 'play down' the structure (e.g. tutor to class), this can be seen as a form of power as it emphasizes the knowledge as power position;

(d) self-disclosure; the use of self-disclosure is important in a group situation as it can promote trust within the group. The leader should not 'splurge' their emotions to create a feeling of 'the more advanced woman', relieving her frustration. Self-disclosure should be used to create a feeling of reciprocal relationships within the group;

(e) leadership and skill; individual leadership is viewed with suspicion by feminist community workers, yet skills are linked with leadership. The worker must strive to develop a form of co-leadership, developing all of the members' skills. This acts as a way to free women from the oppressive hierarchy and allows them to teach and learn from each other;

(f) structure; a structureless group can cause problems, yet an over-structured group can be oppressive in its hierarchy. The group should strive to create a group which is comfortable with the amount/lack of structure (Barker, 1986).

Within women's community groups, these six areas should be

watched and continually modified according to need. The use of these groups by women is often dictated by how comfortable the individual feels within the group and with the worker/leader.

Lack of understanding of women's specificity

Women, as clients, contain members of special needs groups which require special attention. Older women, Aboriginal women, migrant women and lesbians all have special needs not met by existing services, which centre on Anglo-Celtic heterosexual middle-class clients. These assumptions, which bias community and medical services, have negative effects which hinder the use of certain services. Women use medical services more than men and visit medical staff in different capacities for different reasons. Women go as people, who have medical problems, as women who have contraceptive needs, as a chaperone for children and the aged, and as mothers, and pregnant women who have gynaecological needs (Broom, 1988).

Older women suffer from medical staff who do not attempt to find a form of prevention, but who continue to prescribe drugs for all problems. Not all of older women's problems are physical and may be related to arthritis, poor nutrition, old age pains, poverty, loneliness and fear. These problems often are not investigated by local doctors, who try to calm their client through the over-prescription of medication (Curtis, 1986).

Aboriginal and immigrant women suffer from a lack of communication by medical doctors who are not involved with events and circumstances of women's lives. Side effects are often not explained; there is an overwhelming assumption that the client is able to read, and understands the labels on the medication, and is aware of how frequently the medication is to be taken (Curtis, 1986).

Lesbians suffer from the structural problem of the heterosexist society which classes both female and male homosexuality as the same, both deviant and socially unacceptable. The language used can be offensive and causes the service to be lacking (Grant, 1986).

These problems with medical services are compounded by the lack of female doctors. Some women face restricted alliances with men, yet are forced to endure visits to a male doctor. Some women just feel more comfortable with a female doctor. This problem is now addressed through education and social justice policies, yet there is still an over-representation of male doctors in suburban practices. The main assumption (held by some members of the medical profession) is that because women are the carers in society, they can care for themselves. This is not always true, as women generally have so many things to do that their health is often pushed aside, so that they do not let others down (Broom, 1988; Schultz, 1990).

Conclusion

Community care in Australia (i.e. care in the community by female carers) is problematic. Descriptive language is ambiguous as it serves to camouflage the sexual division of labour. A long-term goal of feminism is to transform society (Creed and Tomlinson, 1984); as community care does not question but reinforces cultural stereotypes, it should be the direction of feminist community workers to question the development of community care. The movement of care into the community assumes female labour will always be available (Mowbray and Bryson, 1984). It is assumptions like these which need to be redressed.

If community care is to be a continued aspect of Australian society, strategies should be formulated to support the carers. Moore (1989) has suggested short- and long-term strategies for the development of community care:

Short-term strategies

- Support should be available from the public sector; sexism and discrimination cannot be combated if they are kept in the private sector.
- Anti-discrimination policies should cover people from poverty-related ill health and breakdown.
- Alliances should be developed between carers and care-groups to counter the divisions that result from government policies.
- Democratically accountable needs-based services should be available to provide alternative support for the carers.
- There should be a stop to the stereotyping of aged people as incompetent.

Long-term strategies

- The offering of women a real choice as to whether they wish to be primary carers or not.
- The financial cost of care should be accepted and economic rationalism should be ignored when it comes to the well-being of individuals in society.
- The responsibility of care should be accepted by the governments which are in place to cater for the needs of the state.
- The reconstruction of the labour market and relevant policies to cater for the primary caregiver. This includes the possibility of time-sharing projects and the rejection of the stigma of part-time work as non-valuable.
- There is a need to redefine independence, not in patriarchal terms, but in terms of collective and mutual support.
- Recognition of the community of people as a social group, to be more involved in the planning and practice of such services.

Politicians in Australia have become aware of the importance of women's issues when running for office. The former Labor government began to address issues of discrimination by creating Equal Opportunity units and Affirmative Action policies. A consequence of these is the creation of a National Agenda for women, outlining change and growth projecting to the year 2000 (ABS, 1993c). The policies and strategies in the agenda are only as strong as the individuals who implement them and the access specific groups have to them. While being reasonably comprehensive, the continued lack of participation in the private sphere is noticeable; this relies on the assumption of the availability of a primary caregiver (women) in the private sphere.

Of the two political parties, the Labor Party and the Liberal–National Coalition, the Labor Party has been traditionally for the worker, leaning from the centre-left of the political spectrum. The policies developed by the former Labor government, including privatization policies and the development of community care, is an example of how dissent from the New Right is pervading society. The current Liberal–National government is already undertaking restructuring of industrial relations and education funding; its stand on those previous policies is less than explicit.

References

ABS (Australian Bureau of Statistics) (1992) How Australians spend their time. cat. no. 4153.0.

ABS (Australian Bureau of Statistics) (1993a) Labour Force Statistics. cat. no. 6101.0.

ABS (Australian Bureau of Statistics) (1993b) Women in Australia. cat. no. 4113.0.

ABS (Australian Bureau of Statistics) (1993c) Women shaping and sharing the future: the new national agenda for women 1993–2000.

Baldock, C. (1988) Volunteer work as work: some theoretical considerations. In *Women, Social Welfare and the State* (C. Baldock and B. Cass, eds). Sydney: Allen and Unwin.

Baldwin (1993) *The Myth of Community Care: an Alternative Neighbourhood Model.* London: Chapman and Hall.

Barker, H. (1986) Recapturing sisterhood: a critical look at 'process' in feminist organising and community work. *Critical Social Policy,* 16, 80–90.

Barrett, M. (1980) *Women's Oppression Today.* London: Verso.

Beechey, V. (1987) *Unpaid Work.* London: Verso.

Broom, D. (1988) In sickness and in health: social policy and the control of women. In *Women, Social Welfare and the State* (C. Baldock and B. Cass, eds). Sydney: Allen and Unwin.

Chodorow, N. (1978) *Reproduction of Mothering: Psychoanalysis and the Sociology of Gender.* Berkeley: University of California Press.

Creed, H., Tomlinson, J. (1984) The role of ideology in community work: contributions from feminism and the left. *Australian Journal of Social Issues,* 19, 271–283.

Curtis, Z. (1986) Older women's oppression. *Critical Social Policy,* 16, 109–113.

Delphy, C., Leonard, D. (1992) *Familiar Exploitation: a New Analysis of Marriage in Contemporary Western Societies.* London: Polity Press.

Dolan, J. (1991) *The Feminist Spectator as Critic.* Michigan: University of Michigan Press.

Eisenstein, H. (1984) *Contemporary Feminist Thought.* London: Unwin.

Eisenstein, Z. (1986) *The Radical Future of Liberal Feminism.* Boston: Northeastern University Press.

Grant, J. (1986) Struggling for equal opportunities for lesbians in local services. *Critical Social Policy,* 16, 113–119.

Hartmann, H. (1981) The unhappy marriage of Marxism and feminism: towards a more progressive union. In *Women and Revolution: a Discussion of the Unhappy Marriage of Marxism and Feminism* (L. Sargent, ed.). Boston: South End Press.

Iragaray, L. (1985) *This Sex which is not One* (translated by C. Porter). Ithaca: Cornell University Press.

Kinnear, A., Graycar, A. (1984) Ageing and family dependency. *Australian Journal of Social Issues,* 19(1), 13–26.

Marx, K. (1972) *Marx on the History of his Opinions* (R. Tucker, ed.). The Marx Engels Reader. New York: Norton.

Mowbray, M., Bryson, L. (1984) Women really care. *Australian Journal of Social Issues*, **19**, 261–272.

Moore, S. (1989) Community care of women's work. *Impact*, **19**, 9–12.

Moore, S. (1990) Privatisation at a community level. *Impact*, **20**, 14–15.

Novarra, V. (1980) *Women's Work, Men's Work: the Ambivalence of Equality*. London: Marion Boyars.

Pascall, G. (1986) *Social Policy: a Feminist Analysis*. London: Tavistock Publications.

Schultz, R. (1990). Caring for the caregivers. *Impact*, **19**, 10.

Solanas, V. (1971) *SCUM Manifesto (society for cutting up men)*. London: Olympia.

Tapper, M. (1986) Can a feminist be liberal? *Australasian Journal of Philosophy*, **64** (suppl.), 37–47.

Tong, R. (1989) *Feminist Thought: a Comprehensive Introduction*. London: Routledge.

Townsend, S. (1995) Women and labour. *Australian Feminist Studies*, **22**, 1–8.

Walby, S. (1990) *Theorising Patriarchy*. Oxford: Blackwell.

Young, I. (1981) Beyond the unhappy marriage: a critique of dual systems. In *Women and Revolution* (L. Sargent, ed.). Boston: South End Press.

Chapter 9

Aspects of informal care in Northern Ireland

Eileen Evason

Introduction

Some significant findings from research conducted in Northern Ireland are presented, examining the needs and circumstances of informal carers. The results indicate that, while it might be thought that many of the features of life in Northern Ireland would produce a greater capacity amongst families and neighbourhoods to provide informal care, in practice there is little hard evidence of this. In effect, informal welfare networks have proved as difficult to uncover in Northern Ireland as elsewhere. The data available indicate that, though the context may differ, the needs and circumstances of carers in Northern Ireland, and the cost and consequences of caring, deserve as much attention by practitioners and policy makers there as in the rest of the UK.

Context

It may appear that in Northern Ireland there is a slightly lower need for care and a potentially greater volume of support in the community. The proportion of the population aged over 75 years is the lowest in the UK (Central Statistical Office, 1994) and women in Northern Ireland are less likely to be in paid employment than women in England, Scotland or Wales (Central Statistical Office, 1994). In addition, larger families and the persistence of strong family (and in many areas community) ties might be thought to result in more people being able and willing to share the task of supporting elderly persons and persons with a disability in the community.

This greater potential for the provision of informal care is underpinned by statutory authorities, in a better position, it may be thought, to deliver effective care in the community as a result of the rather different way in which health and welfare services are administered. The region has four appointed Health and Personal Social Services Boards which are responsible for assessing the need for both health and welfare services in their areas, and purchasing the care deemed to be necessary. As in Britain, hospitals may seek trust status but so also may whole units of management which provide non-trust hospitals, and community health and personal social services including childcare.

In assessing the likely impact of these differences, several further points need to be borne in mind, however. First, with regard to the need for care, the lower proportion of very elderly persons in the population is offset by higher levels of disability. As a result of differences in class structure and culture, together with the conflict of the past 25 years and high levels of poverty and unemployment, the prevalence of disability among adults in Northern Ireland is significantly greater than in other UK regions and the level of child disability is slightly higher (McCoy and Smith, 1992; Policy Planning and Research Unit, 1992).

The balance of the caring task is therefore different in Northern Ireland. This may account for the fact that women in Northern Ireland are much more likely to be carers than men. Data from the mid 1980s indicated that, while the proportion of women identifying themselves as carers in Northern Ireland was close to the figure for Britain (14% and 15% respectively), the proportion of men caring was lower, with 9% of male carers in Northern Ireland compared with 12% in Britain (Policy Planning and Research Unit, 1986; Green, 1988). More recent data (Evason and Robinson, 1996) indicate that in 1994 the majority (57%) of informal carers in Northern Ireland were women and, more significantly, that 53% of female carers in Northern Ireland devoted more than 10 hours a week to caring with the corresponding figure for male carers being 29%.

These differences are hardly surprising as male carers tend to be concentrated in one particular caring situation: the care of elderly spouses (Parker, 1990). In contrast, female carers provide support across a much broader range of caring situations. In essence, there is less need in Northern Ireland for the kind of caring that men are most likely to provide, and more need for other forms of care which tend to be undertaken by women. In addition, there is greater adherence to traditional perceptions of male and female roles; local studies indicate caring is defined as women's work (Offer *et al.*, 1988). Thus it seems likely that the volume of care required in Northern Ireland is at least as great as elsewhere, but a heavier proportion of this falls on female carers.

With regard, specifically, to the position of women in Northern Ireland, it cannot be assumed that their weaker attachment to the labour force results in a greater capacity to carry the larger part of the caring task without difficulty. Though declining, the birth rate in Northern Ireland remains higher than elsewhere (Central Statistical Office, 1994) and the region has the least adequate structure of day care facilities for children of any region in the UK (Cohen, 1988). Women in Northern Ireland therefore have heavier family responsibilities and less formal support than elsewhere.

Beyond these issues, there is the question of whether larger families and stronger family and community ties actually result in a larger available pool of informal care. Account must be taken of the very high levels of outward migration from Northern Ireland and the research discussed below indicates that it is not evident that more tightly-knit families and communities result in more sharing of the caring task.

Finally, with regard to Northern Ireland's different structures for providing health and personal social services, the extent to which the potential of integrated administration has been realized in the past has been questioned (Social Services Committee, 1985). Additionally, the recent reorganization of services, which sought to import the concepts underpinning developments in Britain, may have produced a structure which is excessively complex for so small a region and a source of confusion among carers and those needing assistance (Whittington *et al.*, 1994).

On the basis of all of these issues, recent research directly focusing on carers has addressed four main themes. First, there have been attempts to examine the extent to which care is shared across networks of relatives, friends and neighbours (St Leger and Gillespie, 1992; Evason and Whittington, 1992, 1995). Second, there has been some analysis (Evason and Whittington, 1995) of the degree to which carers in Northern Ireland incur the employment, financial and other costs that have been repeatedly documented in British research (Baldwin, 1981, 1985; Joshi, 1987; Ungerson, 1987; Lewis and Meredith, 1988; Parker, 1990; Twigg and Atkin, 1994). Third, some attention has been paid to carers' perception of the adequacy of statutory provision and their views on the appropriate division of labour between the family and the state in the future (Evason and Whittington, 1995). Finally, one small study has sought to address the needs of ex-carers (Evason and Whittington, 1995).

Who cares?

The rhetoric of community care suggests that elderly persons and persons with a disability in the community are able to call on assistance from a range of sources: family, friends and neighbours. However, Parker's (1990) summary of British research suggests that friends and neighbours are not significant sources of support and the extent to which relatives share care is often very limited. In Northern Ireland the small amount of research conducted during the 1980s produced contradictory results. Thus, Burton's (1985) study of the care of children with cystic fibrosis suggested that main carers received substantial help from others; a subsequent study of children with a learning disability (Evason, 1986) indicated that care was overwhelmingly provided by mothers with little assistance from other family members and virtually none from sources outside the family.

The question of exactly who provides what help is particularly important in Northern Ireland as practitioners may bring to their work their own perceptions of the region as a more caring community and exaggerate the volume of informal help available. Two studies conducted between 1991 and 1993 therefore sought to examine the sources and nature of informal care more precisely. The first study (Evason and Whittington, 1992) was of 84 households containing persons requiring care in North Down; the second was of 93 carers in Belfast (Evason and Whittington, 1993, 1995). The first group consisted of persons known to the unit of management in the area. The Belfast carers were drawn from a larger pool (115) of persons known to voluntary organizations and allied bodies in Belfast with the selection of those to be interviewed based on a concern to obtain balanced subsamples of carers across a variety of caring situations.

Both studies produced very similar results, and these are consistent with other work.

The North Down study indicated that where help was required with physical and personal care (for example assisting the person cared for getting into and out of bed and using the toilet), the bulk of the aid required was provided by a main carer. More specifically, 26 of these 84 carers had no help of any kind with physical care, supervision or practical matters such as shopping and cleaning. In addition, among those carers (52%) reporting they received help from other family members, it emerged that in 23 of the 44 families concerned this assistance was confined to watching over or 'keeping an eye on' the person requiring care. Statutory service, rather than neighbours or friends, was the other main source of support.

Building on this, the second study of 93 carers in Belfast sought to quantify the help required and the inputs of those providing care. The volume of help needed was calculated using a points system and these points were then distributed across those who normally assisted with the tasks in question. Two conclusions of significance emerged from this exercise. First, the results indicated that more care was required by those with female carers. Thus, those people with female carers had an average score of 11.6 on the need for personal and physical care while those with male carers scored 9.2. Second, as Table 9.1 indicates, other relatives made a limited contribution to personal and physical support; statutory services were the next most important source of assistance. The findings from these two studies are consistent with much of the data from a study of social networks and caring in three Belfast communities. These results indicated that friends and neighbours played a very small role in physical care and that the size of networks 'has rather limited relevance to receipt of informal help of a practical or task kind' (St Leger and Gillespie, 1992).

Table 9.1 Contributions to caring of main carers and others: % of support provided where required

	Personal care	*Keeping company*	*Tasks, e.g. shopping*
Main carer	71	66	80
Other relatives	16	28	12
Statutory services	10	–	7
Friends/neighbours	–	2	–
Other*	3	4	1
Total	100	100	100

* Mainly privately purchased support

In sum, the data for Northern Ireland indicate that practitioners need to identify precisely how much support is likely to be forthcoming from informal sources other than main carers. The evidence to date suggests that the model underlying much of the debate preceding the restructuring of community care (Griffiths, 1988; DH/DSS/Welsh Office/Scottish HHD, 1989; DHSS (NI), 1990), which placed statutory provision at the margins of networks of persons in the community sharing care, is inappropriate in Northern Ireland.

The costs of caring

The Belfast and North Down studies also examined the costs of caring. The Belfast study suggested that the effect of caring on employment is greater than might be expected in a region with very limited opportunities for paid work; 38% of these carers had left their jobs as a direct result of their caring responsibilities and a further 15% were still in employment but had moved from full-time employment to part-time work. It can be noted that a study in the early 1990s of 1000 women of working age in Northern Ireland found that those with caring responsibilities were less likely to be in full-time employment than those without such responsibilities. The chances of women being in paid employment decreased as the number of hours devoted to caring increased (McLaughlin, 1993).

The Belfast and North Down studies also indicated that caring had a significant impact on the physical and psychological health of these carers. One-third of the North Down carers, for example, reported that their own physical health had deteriorated as a result of the pressures of caring. The results of administering the General Health Questionnaire to the Belfast sample indicated that 34% felt 'unhappy and depressed' and 38% had sleeping problems.

In addition, in both surveys, a significant minority of those interviewed (23% Belfast, 26% North Down), appeared to have very limited social contacts, being visited by relatives or friends once a fortnight or less. Carers will find they have less time to visit; other people may visit carers (and those cared for) less often.

Within the specific context of Northern Ireland, these findings underline the importance of careful assessment rather than assumptions based on broader perceptions of family life in Northern Ireland.

The role of the State

A central objective in the Belfast and North Down studies was to examine carers' perceptions of the quality of the services received. Unmet demands and carers' views on the appropriate division of labour between the family and the State were also measured. In addition, because the Belfast study extended over three years (with carers interviewed at yearly intervals) some attempt was made to assess the impact on these carers, and those cared for, of the 1993 restructuring of provision.

The first set of themes dove-tailed into the concepts underlying the five-year plan for health and personal social services in Northern Ireland for the period 1992 to 1997 (DHSS (NI), 1991). This placed heavy emphasis on targeting of services, implying significant scope for reducing the numbers served, and on improving the quality of provision. Both the North Down and Belfast studies suggested, however, that high levels of satisfaction already existed with the quality of provision and that carers were more likely to be concerned about the quantity of services available.

Thus, in the Belfast study over 90% of those in receipt of four key services (home helps, district nursing, respite care and day centre provision) were 'very' or 'quite' satisfied with the quality of the care offered but levels of satisfaction with the time allocated tended to be lower. In addition, beyond those people wanting more assistance, there were others currently outside the scope of various services who wanted access to them. Demand among the latter group would, if met, have increased the proportion of persons in the study in receipt of, for example, home help and chiropody services by 50% in each case.

Among the 24 Belfast carers who had unsuccessfully sought access to a service, or to an increase in the volume of a service already provided, the outcome was rarely related to the needs of the person cared for. In three instances the service was not provided on the grounds that it would be of no benefit to the person needing care. Six persons had been placed on waiting lists. In the majority of cases (15) rejection related to pressures on provision: 'I was told there just wasn't any more available'; 'I was turned down because of the cutbacks'.

In line with the evidence from Britain (Carers National Association, 1994), there was little evidence of significant improvement as a result of the reorganization of community care. In the year following these changes the carers (37) who participated in the final stage of the Belfast study reported 18 instances where some change had occurred in one of the services received. In the majority (13) of cases, the differences related to decline rather than improvement with hours being cut or the quality of care being affected. In the view of carers, staff seemed to be under more pressure and be more hurried in their work.

More broadly, consultation with major voluntary organizations in the region suggested that the new arrangements were viewed as excessively complex and confusing. The structures for delivering community care differ from Board to Board, as do the titles of key professionals who may be 'care managers' in one area and 'care coordinators' in another. In addition, there is some indication (Whittington *et al.*, 1994) that in Northern Ireland, as in Britain (Twigg and Atkin, 1994), while the costs of the new system are difficult to track, less choice is being delivered with an increase in costs, rather than lower costs and more choice.

With regard to the future the Northern Ireland data draw attention to the danger of the State and families having very different perceptions of their respective responsibilities. In the Belfast study, only 10% of carers thought that in future family members should provide more of the care required by elderly persons and persons with a disability. Only one carer thought that neighbours and friends should 'be encouraged to do more'. Overwhelmingly these carers thought the State should do 'a bit more' (23%) or 'a lot more' (66%). Moreover, with regard to their own specific responsibilities, most carers in both studies assumed the State, not other family members, would take over from them, should care still be required when (or if) they were no longer able to provide support.

Ex-carers

Problems may be encountered by carers when their responsibilities come to an end as a result of the death, or admission to some form of institutional care of the person cared for. They have received relatively limited attention, however (McLaughlin, 1991; Glendinning, 1992). In Northern Ireland the issue has been addressed in only one small exploratory study of 15 ex-carers (Evason and Whittington, 1995). Those interviewed experienced a sharp drop in income when caring ceased. The benefits payable to the person requiring care had typically formed a large part of total household income. Moreover, these ex-carers had often had difficulty negotiating a new identity for themselves with the benefits system. Ex-carers of working age, without wages or spouses to rely on, must redefine themselves as either unemployed and actively seeking work, or unfit for work by virtue of ill health. The difficulties of doing so could leave ex-carers with a sense of being abandoned once they had served their purpose. Five of these women were on invalidity benefit when interviewed; all had to go through appeals procedures to establish their entitlement to this benefit.

The second major theme to emerge from these interviews related specifically to ill health. All of these ex-carers reported significant health problems in the post-caring phase: normally extreme fatigue, accompanied by a variety of other problems, ranging from cancer to agoraphobia. While the majority (nine) of these ex-carers had been in paid employment in the past, only two had returned to work at the time of the interview. Both of these women were in part-time positions. Finally, the loss of the caring role could deepen the social isolation of ex-carers. Most referred to the way in which caring had affected their social lives. The subsequent loss of the relationship with the person cared for, and the contacts arising out of the caring role, could therefore result in an acute sense of loneliness.

The circumstances of these ex-carers are merely suggestive of the difficulties which may arise for those with the heaviest caring responsibilities. There is a need for policy makers and professionals to consider the necessity for a switch in focus and transitional, supportive measures when caring ends. The abrupt withdrawal of support and provision may increase carers' feelings that they have no value outside their utility in delivering 'community care on the cheap'.

Conclusion

Some of the data from the limited number of studies relating to informal care in Northern Ireland have been reviewed. The results of the research undertaken suggest three main conclusions. First, the need for care is probably as great as in Britain but the distribution of caring between men and women is different, with a heavier burden falling on women. Second, it is not apparent that the persistence of strong family and community ties results in more shared care and the costs of caring to main carers in Northern Ireland appear to be as high as anywhere else. Third, statutory provision is the most important source of support after the immediate family. Most carers want this form of provision developed, in preference to greater reliance on alternatives (such as friends and neighbours), and assume the State will step in if they become unable to care. There is clearly a danger of a growing mismatch between the preferences and expectations of carers and the State. Finally, there is a need to devote additional attention to the difficulties which may occur in the post-caring phase – not least, perhaps, because the savings made through reliance on informal care will be reduced if carers subsequently require support.

References

Baldwin, S. N. (1981) The financial consequences of disablement in children: final report. *Social Policy Research Unit, Working Paper DHSS 76*, University of York.

Baldwin, S. N. (1985) *The Costs of Caring*. Routledge and Kegan Paul.

Burton, L. (1985) *The Family Life of Sick Children*. Routledge and Kegan Paul.

Carers National Association (1994) *Community Care: Just a Fairy Tale?* London: Carers National Association.

Central Statistical Office (1994) *Regional Trends 29*. London: HMSO.

Cohen, D. (1988) *Caring for Children: Services and Policies for Child Care and Equal Opportunities in the United Kingdom*. Brussels: Commission of the European Communities.

DH/DSS/Welsh Office/Scottish Office (1989) *Caring for People: Community Care in the Next Decade and Beyond*. London: HMSO.

DHSS (NI) (1986) *Strategic Planning for the Health and Personal Social Services 1987–1992*. Dundonald House.

DHSS (NI) (1990) *People First: Community Care in Northern Ireland in the 1990s*. Belfast: HMSO.

DHSS (NI) (1991) *A Regional Strategy for the Northern Ireland Health and Personal Social Services 1992–1997*. Belfast: Department of Health and Social Services.

Evason, E. (1986) *Mentally Handicapped Persons and Their Families – Who Cares?* Coleraine and District Society for Mentally Handicapped Children and Adults.

Evason, E., Robinson, G. (1996) Informal care in Northern Ireland. In *Social Attitudes in Northern Ireland 1996* (R. Breen, ed.). Belfast: Appletree Press.

Evason, E., Whittington, D. (1992) *Quality and Caring, Centre for Health and Social Research*. Coleraine: University of Ulster.

Evason, E., Whittington, D., Knowles, L. (1993) *The Cost of Caring – First Interim Report of a Longitudinal Study into the Circumstances of Carers in Northern Ireland*. Belfast: Northern Ireland Equal Opportunities Commission.

Evason, E., Whittington, D. (1995) *Caring, Costs and Consequences: Final Report of a Longitudinal Study of Carers in Belfast*. Belfast: Northern Ireland Equal Opportunities Commission Department.

Glendinning, C. (1992) *The Costs of Informal Care: Looking Inside the Household*. London: HMSO.

Green, H. (1988) *1985 General Household Survey Informal Care Report*. London: HMSO.

Griffiths, R. (1988) *Community Care: Agenda for Action*. London: HMSO.

Joshi, H. (1987) The Cost of Caring. In *Women and Poverty* (C. Glendinning and J. Millar, eds). Brighton: Wheatsheaf Books.

Lewis, J., Meredith, B. (1988) *Daughters Who Care: Daughters Caring for Mothers at Home*. London: Routledge.

McCoy, D., Smith, S. M. (1992) *The Prevalence of Disability Among Adults in Northern Ireland*. Belfast: Policy, Planning and Research Unit, Department of Finance and Personnel.

McLaughlin, E. (1991) *Social Security and Community Care: The Case of the Invalid Care Allowance*. Department of Social Security Research Report, no. 4, London: HMSO.

McLaughlin, E. (1993) Informed Care. In *Women's Working Lives* (J. Kremer and P. Montgomery, eds). Belfast: Northern Ireland Equal Opportunities Commission.

Offer, J., St Leger, F., Cecil, R. (1988) *Aspects of Informal Caring: Some Results from a Study of a Small Town in Northern Ireland*. Belfast: Department of Health and Social Services.

Parker, G. (1990) *With Due Care and Attention*. London: Family Policy Studies Centre.

Policy Planning and Research Unit (1986) *Continuous Household Survey Monitor 1/86*. Belfast: Department of Finance and Personnel.

Policy Planning and Research Unit (1992) *The Prevalence of Disability Among Children in Northern Ireland*. Belfast: Department of Finance and Personnel.

Social Services Committee (1985) *Community Care with Special Reference to Adult Mentally Ill and Mentally Handicapped People*. London: HMSO.

St Leger, F., Gillespie, N. (1992) *Informal Welfare in Three Belfast Communities*. Aldershot: Avebury.

Twigg, J., Atkin, K. (1994) *Carers Perceived*. Buckingham: Open University Press.

Ungerson, G. (1987) *Policy is Personal: Sex, Gender and Informal Care*. London: Tavistock.

Whittington, D., Gibson, F., Serplus, B., *et al*. (1994) *Intensive Domiciliary Care Schemes in the Eastern Health and Social Services Board*. Coleraine: Centre for Health and Social Research, University of Ulster.

Chapter 10

Co-creation of pathology: when psychological factors are secondary to socioeconomic factors

Christine Meier and Giorgio Rezzonico

Introduction

The evolution of the sociopsychiatric reality in the Canton Ticino, Switzerland, has been outlined (Meier and Rezzonico, 1990; Monasevic, 1993). There has been a specific move towards community care and rehabilitation, as opposed to institutional care and biological treatment. The present-day situation, however, presents a risk of return to institutionalization, and restrictive methods of social control.

Legislative aspects

Switzerland (6 500 000 inhabitants) is a federation of 26 cantons. Each has a vast legislative autonomy insofar as the Confederation deals solely with matters regarding international relations, national defence and a few others. The Canton Ticino (280 000 inhabitants) differentiates itself from a general Swiss perspective so far as public education and health policies are concerned.

At a legislative level, sociopsychiatric assistance in the Canton Ticino was to be redefined and reorientated after the passing of the 1983 law on sociopsychiatric assistance (LASP) which was intended to be functional by 1985. The priorities dictated by its directives concerned the protection of patients' rights and, in particular, the right to adequate treatment (Borghi, 1978, 1985, 1991, 1992). This was to be interpreted in terms of de-institutionalization and the creation of alternative specialist and personalized services in the community (UTRs).

Article 6 (LASP) states that for an admission to be acceptable, the service and facilities would have to be proportional to the particular need of the patient in question and (where possible), situated in his or her family/social environment. Specialist services would have to be created and, therefore, there would also be a need for on-going staff training schemes. Therapeutic programmes would have to be tailor-made for the individual and, where possible, created in collaboration with the person. A judicial commission would be at the disposal of anybody in need of clarification or legal representation with regard to treatment or admissions (or any intervention which may restrict the patient's personal liberty).

These LASP directives were to substitute the older LISPI directives (law for the social and professional integration of 'invalids'). The LISPI, a law created initially for persons with a physical handicap, had been subsequently applied to sociopsychiatric cases. For persons with sociopsychiatric problems, however, the LISPI directives tended to create chronicity and dependency. LISPI subsidized one's inability to work (a permanent state given a physical loss) rather than funding services focused on prevention and rehabilitation (in the case of a mental breakdown). The irreversibility of a physical handicap (the impossibility of continuing a manual job having lost an arm or leg) may justify the need for a life-time pension. This pension was assigned at a percentage according to the person's incapacity to work due to the handicap (not according to the gravity of the handicap). Such a calculation was not always applicable to a psychological breakdown. The LASP directives would differentiate between the two types of 'handicap' and therefore between the type of intervention necessary.

Organizational tendencies

In 1983 the sociopsychiatric organization of the Canton Ticino (OSC) had divided the territory into three distinct psychiatric sectors which were to include both inpatient and outpatient hospital units for minors, adults and the elderly people. These units, to be known as UTRs (therapeutic-rehabilitative units) would include: outpatient services, consultancy services, crisis-intervention teams in the community, foyers, half-way houses and supervised apartments, psychiatric wards in the general hospitals, single sectors in the Canton's neuropsychiatric hospital and any other service whether public or private which had been authorized by the sector's management and recognized by the LASP.

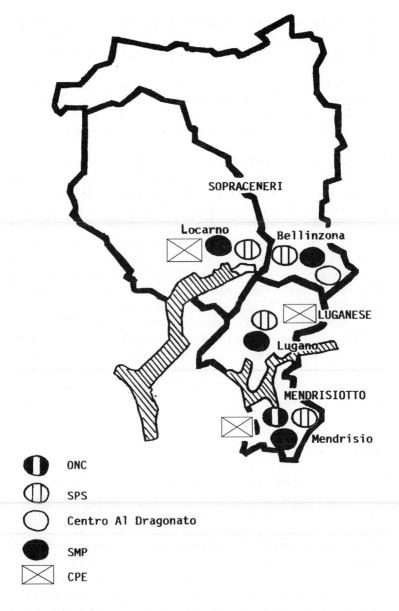

Figure 10.1 Sociopsychiatric organization of the Canton Ticino. ONC–Neuropsychiatric Hospital of the Canton; SPS – Psychosocial Service for Adults; SMP – Medical-Psychological Service for Minors

With regard to the neuropsychiatric hospital of the Canton (ONC) situated at Mendrisio, the law, which it was hoped would promote a tendency towards de-institutionalization, dictated the following:

> The ONC is a place specialized in intense residential treatment. All patients will be guaranteed continuity of care and adequate treatment in their community of origin, designed to avoid the negative implications and consequential dependency characteristic of institutional life.

The three sectors previously mentioned, into which the territory of the Canton Ticino has been divided (Figure 10.1), include the area of Mendrisio (47 000 inhabitants), the area of Lugano (107 000 inhabitants), and the area of Sopraceneri which includes the two areas of Locarno (57 000 inhabitants) and Bellinzona (65 000 inhabitants). The ONC had been divided into the corresponding three sectors, each of which was autonomous in the management of the geriatric and psychiatric wards. Each sector was directed by a psychiatrist who would coordinate the various activities of the already existing Psychosocial Service for adults (SPS), the Medical-Psychological Service for Minors (SMP) and the staff teams for psychogeriatric patients in the community, as well as the sector's various wards in the ONC. By 1985 there would have to be the appropriate UTRs in each sector (private or public) recognized and funded by the LASP. This would gradually decrease the necessity for the ONC as an institutional base in the sector of Mendrisio.

The Foundation Sirio

A particular role was initiated by various private foundations in the creation of alternative community structures (sheltered workshops and apartments, recreation centres), in particular the Foundation Pro Malati, now known as Foundation Sirio (FS). The FS was founded in 1967 on the basis of a donation. Its activities consisted mainly in funding recreational activities for residents in the neuropsychiatric hospital (ONC). In 1984 the FS had started to extend its activity to include rehabilitation, sheltered work and apartments and aimed to promote any new initiative considered worthy in the community. These services were to be created and funded according to the directives of the LASP. Due to bureaucratic and socioeconomic problems, however, these new intermediary structures in the community remained tied and subsidized by the already existing law for the integration of invalids (LISPI). Unlike LASP, they had not the innovative rehabilitative directives which include prevention and personalized treatment.

Nevertheless, the systematic re-organization of the various services commenced in 1984 with the introduction of a rehabilitative programme within the ONC for long-term residents, in particular people with chronic psychotic problems (Rezzonico and Meier, 1987). Based on a cognitive-behaviourist model, the aim was to de-institutionalize and reintegrate these people, by offering them gradual steps towards their community. A 'school' was attended regularly with the gradual introduction of a working schedule (attendance at the two sheltered workshops within the ONC). Group homes and protected apartments were organized (the group home within the ONC and the six protected apartments in the community). A specialized staff team was organized, which included both hospital and community staff. These staff participated in the programme, thus guaranteeing continuity and congruity of care. Above all, familiarity with future caretakers in the community was guaranteed by the staff group prior to discharge.

Where necessary, collaboration and therapy with family and relatives was encouraged. Above all, emphasis was placed on the reciprocal and non-professional support afforded by the group, and on the importance of the working role as a substitute for the sick-role (Meier, 1990). Once in the community, the various group members living together in protected apartments were supervised by the Psychosocial Service for adults. In addition to attending sheltered workshops, they were able to frequent the community Recreation Centre for ex-residents of the ONC. Results from the research carried out parallel to the experience (Meier and Rezzonico, 1992) were used in order to improve methods. The inadequacy of traditional institutional staff training for the de-institutionalization process was evident, necessitating the reconsideration of underlying theoretical models (Meier, Pintus and Rezzonico, 1990).

Five years later: the Centro al Dragonato

After this experience with long-term chronic patients, the FS took interest in a more preventive and needs-based orientation (as indicated by the new sociopsychiatric law LASP). The Therapeutic-Rehabilitative

Centre (Centro al Dragonato) was created for people with more difficult problems, in particular young people with psychotic problems. Rather than de-institutionalize people with chronic problems, the idea was to offer an alternative to hospital admissions by creating the necessary service in the community. Staff would be specialized to deal with the initial (rather than the more chronic) phases of psychotic disturbance (Meier, 1992b).

Created in 1989, the Centro al Dragonato is a non-residential day centre for the social and professional rehabilitation and reintegration of people with both social and psychiatric problems. The inter-disciplinary staff team included both clinical and technical staff. Although initially subsidized by LISPI, the centre was to be one of the first private UTRs, as intended by the new LASP (Meier, 1992a).

Figure 10.2 presents the organizational structure of the centre with the staff relative to each sector.

The on-going staff training programmes include research activity as a prerequisite to a flexible and evaluative approach (Meier et al., 1995). Furthermore, great emphasis is placed on intensive training. There is a conviction that it is the attitude and approach of the staff (their hypotheses as observers (von Foerster, 1981)) that render the Centre's activities therapeutic. The staff team includes non-specialists, with decisions shared by the whole team.

Initial evaluation of client needs is carried out during a 'first encounter' where all significant persons are invited. In this way the needs of all involved may be considered and solutions may be offered comprehensively. The inter-disciplinary staff team with both clinical and non-specialist staff is fundamental. The wide range of services offered, from therapy to jobs and social activity, allows for solutions at all levels (biological, social, psychological). Solutions are personal and continuously evaluated for their effectiveness. Collaboration with all significant persons involved in the situation is constant. Evaluation and intervention is not diagnosis-based (Meier, 1995; Malagoli et al., 1991). The underlying theoretical orientation is constructivist (von Foerster, 1981; von Glaserfeld, 1987; Maturana and Varela, 1987; Burr, 1995).

The *therapeutic centre* works in strict collaboration with the other centres. It serves as an initial reference point for clients and families. Contact is gradually diminished as problems are overcome and more normative relationships are established within the other centres. It has proved therapeutically functional to differentiate between the different services offered at the centre. The *social service*, in addition to dealing with financial problems, collaborates with staff in the various 'sheltered apartments' or 'foyers' in the community, so that objectives and coherency are also maintained at the residential level.

Therapeutic centre	Employment and training centre	Recreation centre
Individual and family encounters for:	Office for the coordination of training and professional activity:	Centre for recreational and cultural activity:
• consultancy/information • evaluation • counselling • psychotherapy • psychiatric treatment	• serigraphy • secretarial work • tailor shop • bar/restaurant • serial work • car mechanics • automatic car wash • gardening • biological agricultural coop.	• bar/restaurant with garden • games room with pool table, pingpong, • library and art club • video/film club • music room
Social service:		
• housing situation • economical situation • welfare		Organization of courses run by professionals
	Job offers	Sport activity
Psychiatric and medical care	Training programmes Apprenticeships	Organization of parties, concerts, tournaments, expositions, dinners, etc.
External consultation	External placements: temporary and permanent	
Including interdisciplinary staff team:		
1 social worker 1 psychotherapist* 1 psychotherapist/psychologist 1 consultant psychiatrist	1 coordinator (employer) 1 graphic artist 1 cook 1 tailor 1 mechanic 1 waiter 1 secretary	1 free time organizer
* Director of the centre	1 horticulturist	

Figure 10.2 Organizational structure of the Centro al Dragonato

The *employment and training centre* offers preparatory courses, apprenticeships and jobs (see Figure 10.2). Unlike a sheltered workshop, it is able to pay realistic wages. Various professionals have been employed (tailor, cook) to supervise the lucrative activities.

The *recreation centre* is open to the young public, thus creating a 'normal' social environment. It organizes various courses and activities both external to the centre as well as through its own facilities (see Figure 10.2).

The Centro al Dragonato is equipped for the necessary research which is carried out continuously and in parallel with all the centre's activities. The centre is experimental, hence it can evaluate continuously the adequacy and validity of services offered. In addition to new methods in the field of therapeutic rehabilitation, the Centre is interested in developing new ideas in the field of sheltered work. These ideas go beyond the traditional sheltered workshop. The Agricultural Cooperative is a step in this direction.

The Centro al Dragonato is situated in the area of Bellinzona in the sector of Sopraceneri, serving a population of 65 000 inhabitants. Its employment centre caters for 60 job requests and an unlimited number of clients are received at the therapeutic and recreation levels. In 1990 it was planned to incorporate it as a service in the OSC. As a model for the other sectors in the Canton Ticino, it would gain its independence from the Foundation Sirio, as one of the first UTRs (whether private or public) as defined by the LASP.

Ten years after: 1994

Results achieved at the Centro al Dragonato have been most encouraging for staff. These staff are convinced that the rehabilitation and integration of persons with psychiatric diagnoses is not an impossible feat. Thanks to the Foundation Sirio, ideas have been put into practice in a most privileged context. However, there remains a paradox: regardless of conscientiousness in improving methods of rehabilitating individuals (and regardless of results in terms of creating autonomous individuals able to cope with their social reality), there seems to be an increasing number of 'invalids' in the Canton Ticino. In addition, these statistics are being used to justify a return to institutionalization and biological methods of social control.

The paradoxical situation is relative to the good results at a therapeutic and rehabilitative level achieved at the Centro al Dragonato. There is apparent non-recognition of this potential at both a legislative/ political and sociopsychiatric level.

The present day paradox was resolved by asking why the move towards community and rehabilitative methods (away from the total institution and restrictive methods) is regarded as a failure. So far there are two clear hypotheses. The first is connected to the socioeconomic/political climate in the Canton Ticino; the second involves the manner in which staff working in the community services have approached this move away from the institution.

Present day incongruences at a legislative/political level

The directive of creating UTRs in the community, subsidized and orientated by the LASP, has only partially been put into function. Partially, insofar as the UTRs which have been recognized by the LASP in the past ten years are those public services which already existed (SMP, SPS, created in 1968). Even the 'day-centres' for recreational activity are supervised by those same public services which tended to offer institutional and biological solutions. There has not, however, been any significant change in methodology or orientation as indicated by the needs-based non-institutional directives.

On the other hand, the Centro al Dragonato (private service), although created under the directives of the LASP, has been 'temporarily' (since 1989) subsidized by the LISPI. It has not been recognized as a LASP UTR even though its methodology is in line with the LASP directives. In this way it is limited in its preventive and non-institutional potential by this less innovative law for 'invalids'.

The process of de-institutionalization and the move towards community care as intended by LASP has been inhibited by the lack of UTRs (as truly intended by the LASP) in the community. As in other countries such as Italy, with its revolutionary 1968 law promoted by Franco Basaglia and his Trieste and Gorizia groups, the ideals represented by the law (Basaglia, 1972), were never put into practice or truly tested. Bureaucratic and administrative problems and the difficulty in significantly changing the institutional approach to a needs-based/community approach in staff have impeded the creation of truly alternative intermediary structures in this field.

On the contrary, de-institutionalization in many areas has resulted in the complete closing down of care services (lack of funds) or the creation of smaller 'institutions' with the same 'institutional' approach being used (lack of staff training, new models of care). Difficulties in effectively transferring funds from institutions to community services are a clear obstacle to successful community care. The lack of appropriate staff training and evaluative methodology in services should not be underestimated either.

With regard to the transfer of funds from institutions to the community, in 1995 funds were invested in Project 2000 (Gambazzi, 1992). Project 2000 has involved the conversion of the ONC (neuropsychiatric hospital) into two distinct sectors. A psychiatric clinic run by medical staff (180 beds) and CARL (a residential centre for the rehabilitation of chronic patients, offering 100 beds, recreation and sheltered employment).

Funds have only been invested in the Mendrisio sector in the above-mentioned 'total institution'. This clearly goes against the directives of the LASP which intended such funding to go towards community services. Paradoxically, ten years ago staff were working towards the de-institutionalization of people with chronic problems from the ONC back into families and communities. From 1995, staff in the socio-psychiatric field will be asked to send them back.

One of the advantages of LASP was that it hoped to overcome certain incongruences of the previous law, LISPI. LISPI was intended to promote the professional integration of clients. For persons with sociopsychiatric problems, the insurance faculty (AI) (and pension for persons considered unable to work due to their invalidity) tended to create chronicity and dependence rather than effectively promote integration. Paradoxically, once labelled with a psychiatric diagnosis such as schizophrenia (considered by many as an irreversible dementia) the person was considered as being incapable for life and given an invalidity pension of roughly SwFr. 1800 (c. £900) a month.

Clearly, this not only encouraged de-motivation; by labelling the person as unable to work, it reduced any possibility of recuperation, creating further emargination and dependency. Other paradoxes were introduced by the AI directives; access to services would be subsidized by LISPI. Where rehabilitation and professional reintegration pro-grammes were possible, a person would have to be considered an AI case and therefore unable to work. Services such as those offered by the Centro al Dragonato have had to deal with this paradox since 1989. Without the AI label clients were not allowed access when motivational levels were still intact. The temptation is often irresistible for young persons with problems who are offered this easy solution (not having to face up to the problems of unemployment, and other obstacles relative to starting from scratch in the professional world). Paradoxically for many young persons in difficulty it would be more successful to fail.

Prevention was thus obstructed by the creation of a condition which furthered invalidity, rather than integration and autonomy. First, chronicity is created by further labelling the individual as 'invalid'. Then centres are required to deal with the problem under the guise of rehabilitation and reintegration when it is possibly too late.

This same paradox will be perpetuated within CARL, whereby services in the community will be unable to cope with a particular crisis (with no true LASP UTRs in the community). Clients will be admitted into the Psychiatric Clinic of Mendrisio; when a situation of chronicity is created, they will then hand their 'chronic patients' over to the total institution CARL where the chances of reintegration and return to normality will be minimal.

Possible hypotheses for the present-day situation

1 At a clinical and rehabilitative level, chronicity is not only an artefact of the total institution where 'madness is manufactured' (Szasz, 1970) but also of the attitudes and approach by staff who often 'bring forth pathology' (Mendez *et al.*, 1988). Psychiatric diagnoses often become alibis for difficulty in finding solutions, failures and relative frustrations (Rezzonico and Meier, 1989). Furthermore, complex problems (which involve individuals, families, staff, institutions, socioeconomic, legislative and ethical aspects) may not be dealt with through a reductionist approach such as found in the medical model (Haley, 1979; Hoffman, 1990; Malagoli *et al.*, 1991). The needs and difficulties of individuals and families go beyond biological perspectives.

   Most of the staff involved in the move from institutional to community care have not received the appropriate training, resulting in pessimistic attitudes and restrictive methods of social control (Haley, 1988).

2 At a political and socioeconomic level, studies in this area (Ciompi 1984; Warner, 1986) have demonstrated how the rise in the number of 'invalids' (or persons with psychiatric diagnoses such as schizophrenia) is proportional in western societies to the rise in unemployment and consequential social stress. Ciompi's research reveals that in countries where unemployment exceeds 5%, rehabilitation and reintegration is improbable. The tendency is to resort to institutional care and biological methods of constraint. Integration is substituted by emargination and social control. In a

society with high levels of unemployment, there is a division between those who work (who are able to achieve gratification and social confirmation within the society) and those people who find themselves in an area of emargination. For the second group there is a need, nevertheless, to guarantee rights and quality of life.

In the Canton Ticino, the recent rise in unemployment has created the usual reactions of individualism, breakdown of solidarity, fear of foreigners and the tendency towards scapegoating. To reduce the statistics revealing increasing unemployment, the first step has been the expulsion of immigrant workers. The second step, in the case of Swiss citizens who may not be expelled so easily from the working world (but who are costly to maintain) may well be to emarginate. By labelling them as 'invalid' they are unable to work, due to mental disorder.

Furthermore, an unemployed person costs the state more than an 'invalid' (an 'invalid' receives SwFr. 1800 maximum). Unemployed persons receive 80% of their normal wage.

This may account for the convenient rise in the number of so-called 'invalids' (defined at an insurance level as persons unable to work). Many may be persons who have simply had difficulty in dealing with the consequences of unemployment/social stress, consequential breakdown, an 'irreversible' psychiatric diagnosis, biological treatment and institutionalization. Thus, the vicious circle is complete. Frustrations in the sociopsychiatric field are justified through the alibi that rehabilitation is impossible for certain irreversible diagnoses. The state offers an easy way out for clients, families and experts, with the invalidity pension. When deterioration is inevitable, the institution is justified as a 'container for rejects'. The checkmate situation is guaranteed by the economic advantage for a society in difficulty (thus creating further emargination, frustration and the need for social control methods).

Possible solutions

Although a 'total institution', a truly rehabilitative approach within CARL may nevertheless promote integration of clients (as opposed to convenient emargination and social control). A time limit is proposed for both clients and the institution, after which clients should be returned to their community. This would impose an approach which looks to the future of the individual as necessarily part of society and not as a social reject.

In addition, to encourage discharge from CARL, UTRs (both private and public) as intended by LASP should be created in all three territorial sectors, both funded and orientated by its directives.

Training schemes and new approaches in community/needs-based care are fundamental to overcome the impotence felt by most experts who have not the necessary rehabilitative training to deal competently with the so-called 'difficult psychiatric cases'. Staff teams should be interdisciplinary, both clinical and technical. Models which are reductionist and methods which are simply restrictive (symptom reduction/social control through chemical lobotomy (Breggin, 1991)) should be substituted by complex and articulate models which aim at needs-based solutions (Meier, 1995).

Research is fundamental at both clinical and administrative levels. The effective benefits of community and rehabilitative care are established, as opposed to institutional and biological methods for clients with psychiatric diagnoses. At an economic level, cost-benefit and cost-efficacy relationships may also be evaluated. Clearly, such an analysis must take into consideration the costs of institutional care (as opposed to community care and effective results of care in terms of increasing autonomy, rather than chronicity). It should also keep in mind the costs of rising unemployment and social stress, which is also alleviated through the creation of institutions for invalids.

If results supported community care (but the secondary benefits are nevertheless superior in the institutional solution), it should be accepted that there are two categories of people; those who can cope and those who are unable to cope. CARL may be developed as the alternative society (B) for those people who cannot cope with society (A). This should occur without creating any illusion of integrating through rehabilitation, and without the need for the alibi of a 'mental disorder'.

Future prospects

There are on-going changes, regardless of the creation of the Psychiatric Clinic and CARL in the territory of Mendrisio. In order to decrease the negative effects of CARL as a total institution, funds have also been used to 'normalize' the grounds where CARL is situated. A well-equipped playground for children and a library/centre for research and documentation have been built in the park, attracting families and students. The ex-ONC's bar/restaurant has been converted, opened to the public and run by waiters (not psychiatric nurses). Technical staff have been employed within the sheltered workshops of CARL and 'stages'/training courses in rehabilitation have been offered to them at the Centro al Dragonato.

Furthermore, there will continue to be a certain investment in the creation of UTRs, recognized and subsidized by the original directives of LASP. In particular, the Centro al Dragonato has been given hope by politicians and administrators in the sociopsychiatric field; by 1998 the centre should be recognized as one of the first private UTRs.

There has been a request by politicians and administrators to carry out a detailed evaluation of the Centro al Dragonato to ascertain cost-benefit and cost-efficacy relationships. This request for a close examination of both methods and costs has been welcomed. The doors of the Centre will willingly be opened to external researchers and evaluators. If successful the Centre will serve as a model for other UTRs.

Also, there have been many requests to formalize at a Cantonal level, the staff training schemes already in practice at the Centro al Dragonato. In 1996 the al Dragonato School of the Foundation Sirio initiated its introductory and biennial courses. Specific training schemes in therapeutic and rehabilitative methods for the reintegration of individuals with psychiatric diagnoses (or serious social problems) have been perfected over the past years. A better understanding of the numerous influences which contribute to crises and breakdown, and the acquisition of strategies and solutions for individuals and families in difficulty, lead to quality treatment. These results promote professional gratification and an optimistic attitude, the best possible prevention against the creation and perpetuation of pathology and chronicity.

References

Basaglia, F. (1972) *Scritti II*. Turin: Einaudi.
Borghi, M. (1978) Per una riforma legislativa. In *Passato, Presente e Prospettive dell'Assistenza Socio-Psichiatrica nel Cantone Ticino* (M. Borghi and E. Gerosa, eds). Bellinzona: DOS, pp. 471–548.
Borghi, M. (1985) *Commento alla Legge Socio-Psichiatrica Ticinese*. Lugano: Bernasconi.

Borghi, M. (1991) *Evaluation de l'Efficacité de la Législation sur la Privation de Liberté à des Fins d'Assistance*. Agno: Pro Mente Sana.

Borghi, M. (1992) *La Legislazione Sociopsichiatrica: un Bilancio*. Fribourg: Editions Universitaires.

Breggin, P. (1991) *Toxic Psychiatry*. New York: St Martin Press.

Burr, V. (1995) *An Introduction to Social Constructionism*. London: Routledge.

Ciompi, L. (1984) Is there really a schizophrenia? The long-term course of psychotic phenomena. *British Journal of Psychiatry*, **145**, 636–640.

Gambazzi, F. (1992) L'Ospedale Neuropsichiatrico del Canton Ticino: Prospettive per gli anni 2000. In *I Percorsi della Riabilitazione* (G. Rezzonico and L. Pintus, eds). Milan: Franco Angeli, pp. 59–72.

Haley, J. (1979) Terapia e controllo sociale. *Terapia Familiare*, **4**, 27–39.

Haley, J. (1988) I diversi modi di valutare la 'schizofrenia' ed i suoi effetti sulle terapie. *Psicobiettivo*, **8**, 49–59.

Hoffman, L. (1990) Constructing realities: an art of lenses. *Family Process*, **29**, 1–12.

Malagoli, M., Togliatti, M., Telfener, U. (1991) *Dall'Individuo al Sistema Manuale di Psicolopatologia Relazionale*. Turin: Bollati Boringhieri.

Maturana, H., Varela, A. (1987) *The Tree of Knowledge: The Biological Roots of Human Understanding*. Boston and London: New Science Library.

Meier, C. (1990) L'inserimento lavorativo come strumento terapeutico nell'integrazione socio-professionale di pazienti definiti cronici. In *Approcci nel Campo della Riabilitazione Lavorativa di Pazienti Psichiatrici in Ticino, I Quaderni OSC*, **8**, 1–58.

Meier, C. (1992a) Il Centro diurno non medicalizzato. In *La Legislazione Sociopsichiatrica: un Bilancio* (M. Borghi, ed.). Fribourg: Editions Universitaires, pp. 217–224.

Meier, C. (1992b) Il Centro al Dragonato. In *Psicoterapia delle Psicosi e Riabilitazione Psichiatrica* (R. Galante, R. Barbarino and L. Viale, eds). San Remo: Servizio Salute Mentale U.S.L. no. 2 pp. 74–86.

Meier, C. (1995) Oltre la diagnosi e verso il cambiamento. In *Nuove Prospettive in Psicoterapia e Modelli Interattivo–Cognitivi* (G. Pagliaro and M. Cesa-Bianchi). Milan: Francoangeli, pp. 231–250.

Meier, C., Rezzonico, G. (1990) Changing outlooks and new directions in psychotherapeutic rehabilitation: organisational tendencies in the Canton Ticino. *Architecture and Behaviour*, **6**, 241–254.

Meier, C., Rezzonico, G. (1992) Risultati di un quinquennio di attività riabilitative con lungodegenti psichiatrici. In *I Percorsi della Riabilitazione* (G. Rezzonico and L. Pintus, eds). Milan: Angeli, pp. 75–102.

Meier, C., Belli, L., Rezzonico, G. (1995) Integrazione sociale e professionale: un progetto di ricera e valutazione nell'ambito di un centro terapeutico-riabilitativo. *Psychoscope*, **6**, 8–10.

Meier C., Pintus, L., Rezzonico, G. (1990) Le modificazioni delle aspettative dell'équipe di un programma riabilitativo come misura del livello di formazione. *Ricerche di Psicologia*, **1**, 95–122.

Mendez, C., Coddou, F., Maturana, H. (1988) The bringing forth of pathology. *Irish Journal of Psychology*, **9**, 144–172.

Monasevic, M. (1993) *L'intervento Psichiatrico nel Ticino*. Lugano: Edizioni

Nuova Critica.

Rezzonico, G., Meier, C. (1987) *La Riabilitazione nell'Assistenza Socio-Psichiatrica: Analisi di una Esperienza.* Milan: Unicopli.

Rezzonico, G., Meier, C. (1989) Un approccio costruttivista al trattamento della schizofrenia: schizofrenia come ipotesi. *Psicobiettivo,* **9**, 35–47.

Szasz, T. (1970) *The Manufacture of Madness.* New York: Dell.

von Foerster, H. (1981) *Observing Systems.* Seaside, CA: Intersystems Publications.

von Glaserfeld, E. (1987) *The Construction of Knowledge.* Seaside CA: Intersystems Publications.

Warner, R. (1986) *Recovery from Schizophrenia: Psychiatry and Political Economy.* London and New York: Routledge and Kegan Paul.

Chapter 11

Psychosocial intervention in nursing: a structural model for holistic care

Gloria Novel

Introduction

The proposed structural model has been developed in order to ensure a specific nursing psychosocial intervention which facilitates a holistic mode of care, in any of the different care situations. First, basic considerations are discussed regarding the nursing profession. Secondly, a definition of the model, its elements and the scope of the psychosocial intervention model are detailed. Finally, a case study is presented to show how it can be implemented in care given to a family member with a terminal illness.

The proposal of a structural model of psychosocial intervention is a basis for care planning, implementation and evaluation, while helping to record the process. The significance is to define a model of intervention. So far as social and psychological aspects of health care are concerned, the model evolved as a consequence of difficulties in listing problems detected in this field. There is also a need to define and plan therapeutic actions to be completed in the psychosocial field. The systematization in the usage of a model of intervention, with its own nursing language, will help in integral care planning. This is also essential to ensure the quality of care supplied by nurses who take care of the person, family or group from a holistic point of view. This involves dealing with the physical, social and psychological aspects (Novel, 1991; Novel *et al.*, 1991).

In addition, this model of intervention starts from a very precise conceptualization of nursing care. The Peplau model of nursing has influenced the psychosocial model, although it is not a conceptual nursing model (Peplau, 1990).

Basic considerations

Nursing as a profession has been defined in various different ways by different authors (Beck *et al.*, 1984; Fernandez and Novel, 1982; Norris *et al.*, 1987; Schoen Johnson, 1993; Wilson and Kneisl, 1992). As a rule, the concepts are not contradictory, but complementary. Following this complementary fashion, nursing may be understood as an *interactional process* between the nurse and the client (person, family or group), in which the *aim is to care*, and the *instrument of care is the relationship* established by the two parties involved.

From this point of view the nurse–client relationship is the core on which all the possible nursing actions are based. 'Care' would be considered to be actions performed by the nurse within a therapeutic relationship. Without this requisite, this performance would be reduced to consider the 'tasks' or 'actions' that could be performed by anyone without the person being a nurse. There are other helping relationships developed by other professionals (solicitors, fire officers) or non-professionals (friends, neighbours, clergy) who are giving support to the person, but with the difference that it is not within a therapeutic relationship. There are no specific therapeutic aims, or other aspects which make the nurse–client relationship unique.

An interpersonal relationship exists in an interaction where each person has a specific effect on the other. This implies support in the maturation, adaptation and integration of life experiences, while helping to find a meaning in the current situation.

Based on this definition, the client–nurse relationship may be conceptualized as a therapeutic relationship, which results in a series of interactions between the nurse and the client for a period of time; a period in which the nurse centres his/her performances on the needs of the person, family or group, by using the knowledge and therapeutic skills which belong to the profession.

The professional relationship aims to provide a solution, or to channel the current problems presented by the patient, family or group, through the therapeutic interventions of counselling and support.

Psychosocial intervention model

The nurse's psychosocial intervention can be defined as: an activity inherent to the process of care, including a number of actions aimed to help the person, family or group:

- to cope with changes and crisis in an adaptative way
- to reinforce the personal resources and
- to transform their vital experiences into elements for personal growth.

The psychosocial intervention, understood in this manner, is carried forward through two kinds of specific actions:

- counselling and
- support.

Counselling includes the actions addressed to supply the client with information, regarding relevant aspects of the health/social and psychological comfort of the person. Another side of nurse counselling is the *teaching* of techniques, processes and methods of self-care and care of others (within the family group). This professional action fulfils the straightforward needs implied in the act itself (information or teaching). It also meets other needs such as security, self-esteem and communication which are fulfilled indirectly.

Support is one of the mainstays of nursing actions. The commonly used term is nevertheless difficult to qualify and quantify. Support can be emotional or material (instrumental). It is necessary to draw a distinction between the two actions:

1 Emotional support is the act of help, motivation and reinforcement, useful to the person's emotional state. This helps the person to bring about necessary changes to adapt themselves to their current problematic situation. Instances of emotional support are to:

- allow and encourage the person to express himself or herself freely about their problematic feelings or thoughts, ensuring the heightened intimacy and confidentiality, in order to promote self-expression
- support the process of personal growth by encouraging behaviour directed to develop self-knowledge and personal competence
- support the change of attitudes towards oneself and others by encouraging and giving alternatives so the person develops new definitions and notions to build up his or her self-esteem
- support the efforts to cope with stressing life experiences by

reinforcing adaptative behaviour and giving feed back and motivational elements when those behaviours are non-adaptative

- support the people belonging to the social network, to help them to cope with their own process of facing stress and at the same time, facilitating their intervention as 'resource-people'.

2 Material or instrumental support is providing the person with the means or elements necessary for him/her to understand a given phenomenon and enabling him/her to set in motion adaptative actions. Examples of material support are to:

- supply elements for the analysis of the current predicament, problematic feelings, thoughts or behaviour, ensuring the necessary feed-back
- help in the search for plausible alternatives, and offering realistic solutions and helping to get them going
- use the person's skills and resources in a therapeutic way within the framework of the nurse–patient relationship, according to its principles
- draw a boundary to the relationship and behaviour of the client or member of a family group, to give the person leeway, in accordance with his or her psychophysical safety
- encourage the active participation of the person or member of the family group into decision-making process regarding their own care and their own life and helping them to set and achieve their personal goals.

Comments on the model

Most nurses carry out some of the activities mentioned above, although a survey of the existing literature would not reveal any record of such activities. One explanation is when interventions are carried out, they usually depend on the nurse's good will. This contradicts the 'process of care' logical methodology where everything is detailed and planned according to therapeutic objectives or results criteria. Nurses express difficulties when trying to register (or when including in the care plan) actions done routinely but intuitively.

To avoid such an intuitive line of work, although it produces results, specific guidelines are required. The activities referring to the 'psychosocial aspects of the care' should:

1 be developed within the nursing process framework
2 come after an assessment of the client (patient, family or group)
3 be set after a nursing diagnosis has been made
4 be in agreement with a care plan established according to the person
   and his or her circumstances.

Following this approach the nurse will ensure the adequate written planning, its implementation and evaluation, for the eventual introduction of corrective mechanisms in the care plan, customary in the job performance. Finally, the systematization of the psychosocial aspects of care responds to the need to make concrete those actions performed with much intuition and self-training.

A case study is presented to show how this model may be put into practice.

Case study: a family with a relative suffering from a terminal illness

This case study involves the family of a terminally ill relative and follows the nursing process steps. The psychosocial intervention model is also presented.

The nuclear family consists of father, mother, a 30-year-old daughter and a 27-year-old son, both married and childless. The family is unable to support sufficiently the terminally ill father, and the nursing team regards them as a subject for care as well.

The 61-year-old father was operated on for a rectal neoplasm, a year before in a second operation. Nowadays, he is semiconscious, he feels confused and his life expectancy is roughly one month. The family was properly informed about the disease's prognosis two years previously.

The process of care

The wife is unable to offer sufficient support to her husband as she herself is dependent to satisfy her needs. For this reason she should be identified as a subject for care.

The daughter and the son present a different need for nursing attention. They cannot offer support to their father because they do not know how to do it. Their demand lies in the lack of knowledge of the subject.

Assessment of basic needs
Dependence/independence data were obtained through interview and observation, according to the assessment guide.

Need for:
a oxygenation: not observed;
b nutrition and hydration: in the last month the wife slimmed. 'She does not feel like eating anything';
c elimination: dependence data are not observed;
d movement and keeping a good posture: since last month the wife spends all day in hospital;
e rest and sleep: the wife finds sleeping difficult;
f wearing proper clothes: dependence data are not observed;
g thermo-regulation: dependence data are not observed;
h hygiene and skin protection: dependence data are not observed;
i preventing danger: independence data – the wife believes that 'the team is treating the patient very well'. The daughter and son's support to the patient and his wife is observed: 'They would like to be useful to both of them', they describe the current situation as one of great importance for them, but they 'try to overcome it';
j communication with others: refusal behaviour is observed on the wife: 'he seems better', 'he recovered from the previous operation, when he felt worse than now. He must have a chance to recover'. Her eyes fill with tears when she talks. Independence data: harmonious relationship with her family;
k living according to their values and beliefs: the wife expresses guilt feelings: she thinks she should have insisted on visiting the doctor earlier: 'In this way maybe we would have spared ourselves so many problems';
l working and fulfilling oneself: the wife feels 'sadness and fury because they were going to retire, they could have stayed with each other and enjoy their free time' (performing the role). She also affirms that she does not feel like doing 'any household job at all';
m playing/participating of recreational activities: the wife spends all day in hospital, unwilling to do anything whatsoever;
n learning: daughter and son ask the nurse: a) about other people's behaviour when they go through such a predicament; b) what is a positive way of helping their parents; and c) if there is in the hospital any professional or system to help their mother and themselves.

Data analysis

Regarding the wife, verbal and non-verbal expressions of suffering occur because of the imminent loss, and negation of the loss, guilt feelings, fury, sadness and lack of energy. These data are the result of an appraisal of the need to communicate, to work and for fulfilment, to play and participate in recreational activities, and consideration of her values and beliefs. Likewise, there was dependence on the nutrition, movement, rest and sleep needs (diagnostic 1).

Certain aspects on the wife's independence data are emphasized: when assessing the need to prevent dangers she seems to rely on the nursing team. Regarding the need to communicate, she maintains a harmonious relationship with her offspring. These data are her own resources to face the stressful situation.

Concerning the daughter and son's need to learn, they show a receptive attitude as they ask for help to improve their knowledge and abilities. They also display an effective and adaptative way to cope with the situation, which makes them 'resource people' for their parents. The siblings describe clearly the situation and its consequences, and their behaviour is focused on objectives of personal growth and help to the rest of their family (diagnostic 2).

Nursing diagnosis

- Anticipatory grieving is due to the imminent loss of a beloved person. It implies negation attitudes, guilt feeling and a careless performance of everyday activities.
- Family coping: potential for growth related to the effective way to approach the situation and the search for a better knowledge of personal resources. Verbally expressed wishes help people learn how to face up to the situation and effectively help their parents.

Commentary to the nursing diagnosis

- Anticipatory grieving can be considered as 'a state in which a person or family experiences feelings of extreme sadness due to the perception of a future loss (of an object, a beloved person or the normal faculties)'.

The difference between 'dysfunctional grieving' and 'anticipatory grieving' is difficult to define; some anticipatory grieving can be considered as dysfunctional grieving. The difference is that with dysfunctional grieving, the loss has already occurred; problems occur because of the way loss and process of mourning is tackled. With

anticipatory grieving the problem appears because the loss (in this case, the husband's death) has not occurred yet; nevertheless, the wife is already behaving like a widow.
- Family coping: potential for growth, is defined as 'the effective handling of adaptative tasks by the family members.

Planning the care

Diagnostic 1

OBJECTIVES

The wife will:
- identify the loss as a future event when talking to a trustworthy person, in four days;
- admit (in the period of four days) the patient's need for support and the possible ways to act, listing in detail how to carry them out;
- identify (in the period of a week) her own needs and look for adaptative ways to live and relate to others, lessening the dependence factors she is currently undergoing.

NURSING INTERVENTIONS*

Counselling activities:
- endeavour to secure the nursing team's continuity so that the wife relies on it, informing her of any change so as to strengthen her confidence;
- inform the wife honestly about the situation, keeping room for hope, emphasizing the aspects that improve the patient's welfare (decrease of the patient's conscious perception of pain, the fact of counting on the support and company offered by her daughter, son and herself);
- contribute with objective and realistic information about the loss and the process of mourning, together with the most effective ways to solve it;
- supply her with information concerning her own physical additional needs, as a consequence of the difficult time she is going through, and the efficient ways to fulfil such needs (not eating

---

*It is both in this part of Nursing Interventions and in the following one (Diagnostic 2), where the Psychosocial Intervention Nursing Model is applied.

alone, going out of the hospital, relating to other people, carrying out some physical exercise, practising relaxation or breathing techniques to get a better rest);

- explain to her the importance (both for the husband and herself) about
  - playing an active role in the care
  - using physical contact (touch and caress him)
  - demonstrating her affection/love
  - talking to him about subjects interesting for both and establishing an effective communication that will comfort both of them.

Support activities:

- guarantee a helpful relationship that allows the expression of the person's problematic thoughts and feelings;
- provide her with the necessary elements for the analysis of the situation that will enable her to understand her feelings regarding the future loss and consider them as normal;
- help her to identify the stage of mourning she is going through;
- help her to cope with the 'negation reaction', avoiding reinforcing it;
- encourage her to analyse her guilt feelings by confronting them with her present helpful and positive actions;
- encourage her to take realistic decisions regarding the near future and according to the resources she has at her disposal;
- identify the personal resources she has available to ensure an efficient coping. Do the same with the social resources of support (offspring, friends and other social network);
- foster her active participation on the care of the husband (involving her in the decision making regarding the care, daily contact, asking her to participate in the routine care);
- offer her the possibility to get the spiritual assistance that she and her husband may feel in need of when taking into consideration their values and beliefs.

Results criteria:

- the wife is able to talk to her daughter/the nurse about her husband's current state. She also expresses the thoughts and feelings derived from the situation;

- she proves herself efficient in taking care and supporting her husband, which makes her feel satisfied;
- The wife begins to take into consideration both her own nourishment, rest, activity and sleep and her personal life and relationships.

Diagnostic 2

OBJECTIVES

The offspring will:

- choose (in the period of four days) the personal resources available to cope with the situation in an adaptive way;
- make use (in the period of a week) of the social and personal resources at their disposal in order to become an element to provide support to the family group;
- provide (at any moment) specific support to the mother with the aim of helping her to cope with the situation in such a way that she manifests feeling accompanied and understood.

NURSING INTERVENTIONS

Counselling activities:

- provide them with information about the resources of support available in the hospital and in the social network (associations, support professionals, etc.) enabling them to take the decision they consider appropriate;
- supply the offspring with objective and realistic information about the situation and vital experiences of their parents, and also about the most effective way to act;
- provide the necessary feed-back to improve behaviours leading to the search for and acceptance of mutual support.

Support activities:

- establish and maintain a helpful relationship and a therapeutic atmosphere of support;
- reinforce positively attitudes of active coping, previously shown;
- guarantee moments of intimacy to encourage the dialogue among the family members;
- support the decision to talk to their mother about the need to plan the future together, according to the forthcoming situation.

Results criteria:
- the daughter and the son feel happy about their acquired knowledge regarding help and support;
- the family members are now able to share their thoughts and feelings and to comfort themselves;
- the mother feels supported and understood by her daughter and son. This fact will help her to overcome the situation.

References

Beck, C. M., Rawlins, R. P., Williams, S. R. (1984) *Mental Health Psychiatric Nursing.* St Louis: C.V. Mosby Company.

Fernández, C., y Novel, G. (1982) *El Proveso de Atención de Enfermería: Estudio de Casos.* Barcelona: Salvat.

Norris, J., Connell, M. K., Stockard, S., Ehrart, P. M., Newton, G. R. (1987) *Mental Health Psychiatric Nursing.* New York: John Wiley.

Novel, G., Lluch, M. T., Miguel, M. D. (1991) *Enfermería Psicosocial II.* Barcelona: Masson-Salvat.

Novel, G. (1991) Hacia una sistematización de los cuidados de enfermería. *Notas de Enfermería,* 3, 155–161.

Peplau, H. (1990) *Relaciones Interpersonales en Enfermería.* Barcelona: Salvat.

Schoen Johnson, B. (1993) Adaptation and Growth. *Psychiatric Mental Health Nursing.* Philadelphia: J.B. Lippincott Company.

Wilson, H. S., Kneisl, C. R. (1992) Psychiatric Nursing, 4th edn. Redwood City: Addison-Wesley Publishing Company.

Chapter 12

Slovene mental health services

David Brandon and Vito Flaker

Introduction

Slovenia is a small country – half the size of Switzerland – situated to the east of Italy, to the south of Austria and to the north-west of Croatia. It has just over two million people. It has a long history, mainly in recent centuries as part of the Austria-Hungarian empire. In June 1991, it broke away from the former republic of Yugoslavia, and after a brief war, formed an independent separate state with Ljubljana as its capital.

It is difficult to see clearly how these massive changes in its status will affect the organization of health and social services. The change from a 'command' to a 'market' economy is taking place rapidly. Increasingly, commercial companies have taken over full responsibility for their own success or failure in a very difficult economic climate. As well as the European and world recession, Slovenians have to contend with the loss of major export markets in the former Yugoslavia, amounting to 50% of the total.

Svetlik (1993) comments that:

> the widespread network of health care institutions has become bureaucratic, fragmented and very expensive. Neither the providers nor the patients are motivated to seek economic efficiency. Vested interests prevent the necessary reforms. As a consequence, expertise and technology lag behind. Low salaries of medical personnel do not motivate good work and the quality of services deteriorates.

This has very serious consequences for the mental health services.

History of Slovene mental health services

The history of Slovene mental health services is not so different from mainstream Europe. Asylums were developed in the nineteenth century, and increased in influence and size. They helped to symbolize the marginalization and stigmatization of the 'pauper lunatics'. People who became mentally disordered were increasingly feared, and then incarcerated. During the Second World War the entire population of Novo Celje mental hospital (430 people) was liquidated in the Nazi euthanasia programme. By 1952, the increasing numbers of hospital patients meant that former castles and barracks were commandeered to use as makeshift asylums.

The 1960s and 70s were a dynamic period. There were direct connections with the radical Basaglia group in Italy. Questions were asked about the politically repressive nature of much of Slovene psychiatry. This resulted in the gradual opening of some hospital doors; an increased questioning about the use of compulsory admissions; a more respectful attitude to patients; some therapeutic communities; rehabilitation programmes; work on prevention, especially in the area of suicide attempts.

Experience of the services

Little of that heady dynamism remains. Longer-stay patients are still mainly in large institutions – some in castles in remote mountain areas. Community care is relatively scarce and underfunded. There have been few developments in the voluntary and private sector while the state had a virtual monopoly under the socialist system. The few innovations were usually small-scale, often initiated through social work, and considered marginal. For example there is a Committee for Social Protection of Madness (now known as ALTRA) inspired, in part, by the anti-psychiatry tradition. It campaigned against bad conditions in some remote institutions and tried to develop small-scale alternatives.

Experiences of service users were often bleak. A Slovene patient with considerable hospital experience wrote: 'The first thing one notices is an out-of-place building which reminds one of a neglected castle. Most of the mental hospitals in Slovenia are parted from the ordinary life... Most frequently they put you in the 'closed department'... where you are usually sharing everything with about twelve other women' (Mike, 1993, personal communication).

Another user commented: 'In the whole five months hospitalization, I have hardly seen "my psychiatrist". Mostly it was during his brief visits on the ward ... enough though to teach me how to hide my problems and act "cool" in order to get out as soon as possible ... The most rewarding experience was to meet other "crazy people". I learned that most of them are very interesting people who have a lot to say' (Mike, 1993).

Paradoxically, this gross alienation and experience of empty space fostered some genuine camaraderie and self-help. Unfortunately, this has been restricted to the hospitalization periods as there are no means of extending it into the community. An ex-patient, now an activist in the users' movement, writes: 'We all know that there is something wrong with what they do to us, that this is not really treatment and doesn't help, even damages us... There was obviously something that went wrong in our lives, but there was nowhere else to go (or to be sent to). Most of us have a notion that things could be done differently but till now we didn't have an idea what this could look like' (Flaker, 1993).

Contemporary Slovenian services

Like any country, Slovenia has a number of mental health problems. It has one of the highest suicide rates in the world: 30 per 100 000 population, which are mostly male deaths. It has a large alcohol problem, and there is also much incipient racism. Currently it offers refuge to about 30 000 survivors from the Yugoslav war – most are Bosnian Muslims. A minority of those (30%) are confined to the refugee camps. It is very difficult for non-Slovenes of any kind to gain acceptance in a mainstream culture which regards them as inferior.

The democratization of Slovene society has some impact on general psychiatry, which historically has been authoritarian. Since independence, there has been a greater willingness among the professions to discuss community alternatives. However, this is not yet reflected in the services nor in funding. Genuine community-based services are still fairly scarce. Current political uncertainties seem to freeze action. Inflation, rising poverty, unemployment and the great influx of refugees (now more than 3% of the population) make it much more difficult to include those people who have always been marginalized both socially and economically.

There is no specific mental health legislation although ALTRA is pressing for a new Act. Although the largest proportion of disabled people in Slovenia are disabled on mental health grounds, legal provision is overwhelmingly tailored to meet the needs of physically disabled people. The whole system of safe-guarding patients' rights is designed badly; it provides formal and legal cover for detention, more than for protection. Since all admissions to psychiatric hospitals are through a closed admission ward, any court trying to safeguard such rights would be flooded with requests for detention orders. Most would be irrelevant as the majority move to an open ward in a day or two.

An attempt has been made to define the essential rights of psychiatric patients. The first advocacy work in Polje Hospital has shown that legal procedures are not followed properly. The court is not notified at the right time; the necessary grounds for compulsory hospitalization are not observed. The Advocacy Group started in the autumn of 1992. During the following year, they intervened in some cases. They also started a band which sang of the misery of mental patients. The group also edited a special issue of the *Journal for Social Work*, worked on legal issues and trained advocates. Their initial efforts were met by defensiveness from the psychiatric authorities. By January 1994, they were operating more fully. The response from users was greater than expected. The majority wanted help with family and employment matters. So far, few complaints have been made about hospitalization and abuses of rights.

Current services

There are six psychiatric hospitals with a total of 1614 beds with an average hospitalization period of 49 days. This total inpatient population is not a true reflection of the actual numbers. In addition, there are psychiatric dispensaries or specialist outpatient departments located in all regions. There are also a number of other institutions, not labelled mental hospitals, of generally even poorer quality; these services house a mixture of elderly, confused people, people with a mental disorder, and people with an intellectual disability. These services include the infamous Hrastovec, housed in a remote castle near Maribor with more than 700 beds, sometimes called the 'Slovene Leros'. In 1985, 43% of the population of old people's homes were diagnosed as mentally disordered.

The largest designated proper mental hospital is Polje just outside Ljubljana with 470 patients. It is grim and bare. Many patients wander around in pyjamas and dressing gowns both inside and outside the main buildings. Half the total population consists of psychogeriatric patients. There is roughly an equal number of men and women patients who are strictly segregated by gender. Six of the 20 wards are secure facilities.

Most new admissions come through the closed wards where they are strictly controlled. Nets are often used to confine patients. Strong nets are tied to the bunk bed frames so that patients cannot get out. Twenty-five per cent of patients are recorded as compulsorily admitted. Some patients recorded as voluntary admissions are threatened with compulsory admission unless they agree to come involuntarily.

A typical ward has 25–30 patients. The daily life is extremely boring. There is a senior nurse in charge who is trained in psychiatry, after taking a general nursing qualification. There are three to four junior nurses plus a cleaner, with a night nurse covering two wards. The ward is largely 'owned' and worked on by psychiatrists. There are very few staff, so very little time can be spent with patients. Much energy goes into discipline and in getting patients to comply with daily routines and disciplines. Some other professionals such as music therapists and psychologists visit and work on the wards. There is little use of social work. Polje has no volunteers although some organizations have offered assistance. Senior medical staff insist that 'it might interfere with the medical work'.

Senior psychiatrists make the major decisions in these hospitals with only token consultation. They control the training of most other professionals. Nurses in the mental health field have extremely low status and little influence. All wear uniforms. Their salary is not enough to afford a reasonable flat and food so they find it hard to live independently from their families. Polje has the money but cannot recruit and keep staff. Nurses leave to train in careers like occupational therapy or emigrate to Austria and Germany, where they can get much more money. There is little community-based psychiatric nursing. Treatment is mostly medication with a little psychodrama and music therapy. The whole atmosphere is very unstimulating.

These sorts of traditional institutions raise fundamental questions about the nature of professionalism. Is it possible for the 'para-medical professions' to gain more influence in making decisions and in the development of different treatments? Currently they are dominated and often crushed by medicine, so they must struggle hard to establish any sort of separate identity. This makes it difficult to develop a diversity of approaches and treatments.

Another serious question is about the relationship between intellectual concepts and everyday practice. This reflects deep schisms in Slovene culture between theory and implementation. There is a strong emphasis on understanding and reflection, rather than on the acquisition of relevant skills. Traditionally, the training in the various professions (especially in social work) has been largely theoretical, with little weight placed on practice and implementation. There is also an absence (apart from medicine) of adequate supervisory systems in which senior practitioners help newly-qualified Staff to improve. The creation and maintenance of good practice thus does not occur. In these circumstances, it is difficult to see how the service outcomes for users can be substantially changed and improved.

There are several important initiatives in the mental health field. A mental health unit in Ljubljana city centre offers groupwork based on psychoanalytic principles. It also has crisis centre facilities with some beds. Many patients can come for day services without staying overnight. There is a great variety of treatments in a much less oppressive atmosphere than at Polje Hospital. However, it is still rather dark and clinical.

Some group homes have been opened for former Polje patients in Ljubljana by some hospital staff. This is linked with some work and activity schemes. The development of community facilities is very slow and piecemeal and meets some opposition. Some English material on relevant practice has been translated and seems to circulate well (Brandon, 1992).

The EC Tempus programme (developed jointly with the English, Italians and Austrians) offers indigenous professionals some post-qualification training in different mental health systems, as well as close contact with foreign academic staff. Ten Tempus students spent six months in the first half of 1993, in various social work, educational and psychiatric placements in London, linked with the Richmond Fellowship, MIND and the London School of Economics; another twelve went to Trieste and one to Austria. A variety of practical initiatives are developing.

ALTRA opened the first Slovene group home for psychiatric patients in May 1992. A network organization for patients meets weekly. The Committee has also developed links with three lawyers to develop advocacy for hospital patients and to press for revision of the mental health legislation. A club is also growing which hopes to develop employment cooperatives like those in Trieste. Another voluntary organization, SENT, pioneers community-based facilities including sheltered work.

Counselling and support services are also growing. The best developed in social services is family counselling and therapy linked with the university. There are support groups for Bosnian rape victims. There is the development of alcohol groups, some linked with Alcoholics Anonymous. It is often hard to get long-term finance for such groups, but many get EC funding, especially PHARE (Poland and Hungary Assistance for Economic Restructuring).

The issues of women in the mental health service have only recently become recognized. In 1988 a helpline for battered women and children began. A women's counselling centre and a shelter are planned. A new study has examined a wide number of important issues in the field of women and mental health in the Slovenian context (Zavirsek, 1993). There is also a development of crisis support as an alternative to hospital admission (Zavirsek, 1996).

Overview

It is necessary (but very difficult) to develop the whole voluntary sector, not seen as important before the establishment of the new Republic. Traditions of volunteer effort and partnership with various professionals which are long-established in many European countries need urgent work. This is one aspect of pluralization (Svetlik, 1993). In the move from state responsibility for poverty and pensions towards rather more individual responsibility, the development of a concentrated network of mutual help and care is vital. Self-help and voluntary activity, however, can never be the same in a Catholic country in central Europe as in a Protestant country in western Europe. The relationship between the individual and the State is fundamentally different, reflecting the whole culture of conscience, particularly around the practice of confession. In Catholic countries, the fundamental question is not 'how to confront the State' but 'how to get around its power and influence'. The questions of so-called socialist influences in the former Yugoslavia have tended to overshadow the powerful religious influences.

Some obstacles to the growth of a vigorous voluntary sector lie in the more technical area. There are substantial fiscal and legal problems. For example, there has been no great tradition of fund-raising which must be learned from scratch. People looked to the State for most social and economic support. Growth of voluntary organizations and mutual support groups is required. Deep changes in the economy and social security system are also required, which involve fundamental issues like decentralization and privatization. But there are dangers that the 'Welfare State' will become primarily the responsibility of the voluntary and private sector rather than an essential and primary responsibility of national government.

Such a dynamic situation leaves spaces for new syntheses and innovation, as well as considerable uncertainties and confusion. For example, the whole field of community care is waiting for development. There is a danger of cultural imperialism, that powerful professionalized vested interests will move in and take over. Slovene psychiatry, in particular, is power hungry and extremely resistant to any radical changes.

Ways forward

The Tempus programme is crucial in this change. These students (many important and influential figures in the Slovene mental health movement) are torn between the seductive and sometimes enchanting realities of Italian/British practices, and the grim realities of the current Slovene mental health services. This is hard to bear both emotionally and ideologically. The challenge lies in fostering grassroots movements. Slovene ways of changing institutional services are required.

A number of important themes emerge from attempts to improve the psychiatric services:

- work on ways to *reduce the stigmatization* of mental patients: the role of the Slovene media could be extensive. There is a great need for positive magazine articles, TV and radio programmes which stress the achievement of patients and former patients. It is also necessary to move away from congregated services like Polje hospital and many others, which tend to magnify stigma, towards more invisible services;
- *increase choices:* lowering the proportion of compulsorily-admitted patients, offering more diverse treatments and much more control by patients; more treatment from home rather than admissions to hospital; greater involvement of social work and the

establishment of community nursing with relevant courses. This would involve the development of a new legislative framework, borrowing from the best in Europe, which stresses the rights of patients and the importance of relevant advocacy;

- *less authoritarianism:* reduce the considerable authoritarian role of psychiatrists; working towards a more enlightened professionalism which shows more humanity of professionals. It is important in this context to challenge the use of psychoanalytic theory as a basis for work as it encourages Slovene professionals to become psychiatric partisans, hiding in psychodynamic mountains;

- *increase the status of nurses:* morale among psychiatric nurses is very low. It is virtually impossible to be serious about improvements in services unless they feel better and more secure about their future. That must involve considerably improved salaries; conditions of service; career structure; and more room for independent decision making. There is an urgent need to develop and provide training in the theory and skills of community-based nursing;

- *establishing effective supervision:* almost all professions, except for medicine, have no system of supervision of the daily practice of trained professionals. Mentoring systems are almost unknown. Quality of service delivery demands that such a system be developed;

- *strengthening the voluntary sector:* Slovenia has an embryonic voluntary movement, for example the Association of Mental Health, Alpe (Adria) which is small but healthy. It needs much more encouragement and financial investment. This should be linked closely with the emerging patients' movement, avoiding the worst excesses of middle class paternalism;

- *encouraging the service user movement:* the basis of fine service always lies in sensitivity to dynamic user feed-back; there are virtually no such feed-back systems in any Slovene services. They need to be developed speedily;

- *translating and writing more practical texts for professionals, service users and families:* some German and English texts would help; but much more Slovene research and writing needs to be completed which is very practical. There is a need for more pragmatic publication materials to encourage the linking of good practice with enlightened theory. Presently these materials are in very short supply.

In general, there are very considerable grounds for optimism in Slovenia. The current quality of psychiatric services is quite poor and although there is a very sophisticated knowledge of European and American services, especially among senior staff, little of this knowledge influences the existing practice. But there is growing awareness of different and complementary therapies in a culture which is very open to New Age materials. There is an honest struggle to establish a tradition of advocacy against much bitter professional resistance. There is also the development of some vigorous voluntary organizations like ALTRA and SENT which pioneer truly community-based facilities but are starved of monies and influence and work their way through many diverse organizational problems. There is also an increasing and important awareness in government that institutional forms of service provision are relatively expensive. Slovene attempts to join the EC must involve the development of more community-based services.

References

Brandon, D. (1992) 'Prakticni Prirocnik – za osebje v sluzbah za ljudi s posebnimi potrebami' Visoka sola za socialno delo, Pedagoska fakulteta, Ljubljana.

Flaker, V. (1993) Nacrtovanje razvoja psihosocialnih sluzb na podiagi potreb Ijudi z dolgotrajnimi psihosocialnimi stiskami na podrocju R Slovenije, fazno raziskovaino porocilo, Ljubljana: Visoka sola za socialno delo.

Svetlik, I. (1993) Reform of social policy in Slovenia: a soft approach. *Journal of European Social Policy*, **13**, 195–203.

Zavirsek, D. (1993) 'Zenske in Dusevno zdravje'. Ljubljana: Visoka Sola za Socialno Delo.

Zavirsek, D. (1996) Crisis support in Slovenia. *Breakthrough*, **1**(1), 11–22.

Chapter 13

Care of people with chronic mental disorders: a European–American perspective*

John Talbott

Introduction

First, there is not really yet a Europe, in the same sense as the Americans think of the USA. So it is really unwise to speak of Europe, or even Western or Central Europe. Second, it is sometimes even difficult to talk of something French (Braudel, 1986) or British, or especially Italian, because local differences are so great, despite single national funding and administrative systems. Third, Central Europe presents even greater problems, given the different histories revealed by such terms as the Prague Spring, Velvet Revolution, Goulash Communism and Solidarity. Especially for those from countries other than the USA there are no universal generalities, and lots of exceptions. However, in this chapter I will attempt to draw some broad similarities and differences between and among countries.

Similarities

Homelessness

Homelessness (and especially homeless people with mental disorders) is now a worldwide problem, no longer the subject of despair only in the USA. In France, the problem is increasingly obvious, a situation totally different from 20 or 10 or even 5 years ago. In Paris it is now estimated that 1% of the population is homeless and a recent headline stated that 'Vagrants Spark[ed an] Orly Strike'. In the UK there is a story each day in the press about the homeless, who are often spoken of

* Original paper presented at Schizophrenia 1992: Poised for Change, Vancouver, BC, Canada, July 19–22, 1992.

semi-romantically as 'sleeping rough'. After further reading, however, their condition is more closely attributed to the 'closing of mental hospitals' and having 'been thrown out into the streets' after discharge. Homelessness is even reported in Japan, Switzerland and Germany despite their astoundingly successful economic progress. In Central Europe, the recent appearance of homeless individuals with mental disorder is attributed (Freeman and Henderson, 1991) to the end of the socialist principle of 'jobs and homes for everyone, no matter how disabled' (the factory's role has even been nostalgically described as partly a community support programme) and to the demise of central planning that looked out for everyone, no matter how vulnerable (Bennett and Freeman, 1991). In the USA a study revealed that 80% of men in a New York shelter suffered from alcohol and/or drug abuse; another survey revealed that Americans are no longer shocked and outraged by the plight of the homeless. In both Europe and the USA, then, there is neither enough basic inexpensive housing, nor enough supportive housing alternatives.

Going from asylum hospitals to community care

The intent of most Governmental leadership in mental health is to move from asylum hospital care to community services. In Central Europe, several countries are rapidly but thoughtfully attempting to put together plans for changing their entire service systems. This change, however, is taking place in the face of tremendous economic problems and pressure to pursue other priorities, making many people fear that such a shift, in the absence of support, will result in American-style 'dumping'. In addition, there is a paucity of trained professionals (including nurses and social workers), a lack of knowledge of all but biological treatment, and a 50-year tradition of central planning rather than local responsibility. However, plans continue with great enthusiasm, intelligence and dedication. European planners desperately want to know: how many of each community services are needed – from general hospital beds to outpatient slots to rehabilitation placements; how many staff are needed; how services fit together and how elements coordinate smoothly.

Focus on people with chronic mental disorder

European Health Ministers have decided to focus on comprehensive care of people with mental disorders; their mental health committee has directed its work to the chronically ill (Freeman and Henderson, 1991). In Central Europe, there is an intriguing wrinkle to this focus, since after 50 years of emphasis on biological and Pavlovian treatment, there is an enormous hunger among practitioners, trainees and even medical students in learning about applying psychoanalytic and psychotherapeutic practice, which for so many years was forbidden and indeed illegal.

Treatments

Three themes dominate: (a) the sophistication and knowledge regarding psychopharmacology, even outside the Czech Republic, long an innovator in psychopharmacological agents, and the resurgence of interest in clozapine, stimulated by recent enthusiasm for the drug in the USA; (b) the respect for and interest in psychosocial approaches and rehabilitation; (c) the interest in integrating pharmacological and psychosocial treatments and rehabilitation, but also by; (d) the desire to know which treatments work for which patients and in what order of priority they should be applied.

Funding

No one admits to adequate funding; indeed, while funding problems may differ in origin, staff complain of: (a) simply not enough money for psychiatric services; (b) lack of parity *vis à vis* funding for other medical services; (c) great tension over national funding priorities (e.g. with other medical, social and development needs, especially in Central Europe); and (d) the problem integrating funding streams (Hurst 1991).

Ideology rather than science propelling change

While more evident in Central Europe, there is a fear of having traded in one ideological basis for operating services (e.g. communism or socialism) for another (e.g. de-institutionalization or privatization). There is a great wish on the part of the leadership to base decisions for future services on scientific data rather than ideology, after realizing how much their prior ideology bankrupted their entire array of operations.

Lack of integration

The fragmentation of services is a familiar hobgoblin to Americans and its causation often attributed almost entirely to the inefficient administrative and funding systems; it is startling to find its occurrence elsewhere. The fragmentation of services in Canada (Wasylenki *et al.*, 1992) and lack of integration at the clinicians' level in the UK (Sim, 1991) have parallels in the USA.

Families

While at very different stages, there is widespread palpable interest in family/patient/ex-patient organizations. Linked to this are a growing number of national Awareness Weeks, a direct result of new or increasingly effective professional–relation alliances.

Differences

Central Europe

Funding
With their economies in absolute bankruptcy, Central European leaders are wary of promoting any steps that look costly. They know that some 'double-funding' is necessary to move from asylum to a more balanced community care system, and are concerned lest this inadequate funding result in *de-facto* 'dumping' as in North America, which embarked on de-institutionalization with so many more resources. Privatization is seen as a solution to some problems (e.g. funding by drug companies of some studies or laboratories and foreign investment in hospitals).

Great asylum/general hospital bed disparity
While subject to all the caveats of over-generalization, there appears to be greater disparity between bed capacity in asylums and the psychiatric units of general hospitals than elsewhere.

Strong psychopharmacological–weak psychosocial capacity
This includes a psychosocial rehabilitation focus based on prior ideology.

Education
There is little formal psychiatric postgraduate training; one observer described how nursing schools were 'destroyed' by the communist regime, and a paucity (if not absolute absence) of trained social workers.

Western Europe

Lack of data
There is a lack of data about the numbers of beds, services provided, as well as a dependence on the same data base mainly from USA studies, with some UK/Scandinavian studies, regarding clinical and services research (Bennett and Freeman, 1991; Freeman and Henderson, 1991). One benefit, however, is that this can lead to utilization by others of already painfully worked-out instruments, forms and scales.

Nationalism, ethno-centrism and other centrism
Despite North American views about Europe, the problems of nationalism and ethno-centrism are threatening not only the former Iron Curtain countries, but other countries; even France and the UK have their own separatist movements, both violent and non-violent.

Distrust of research from elsewhere
There is distrust on the part of some Western Europeans of data from researchers from countries other than 'their own'. Whether such research deals with smoking or antipsychotic efficacy, this distrust leads to duplication and wasted effort.

USA

No national health plan
Of all the industrialized nations, except South Africa, the USA remains the sole hold-out.

Unique legal onslaught
On involuntary commitment and the right to refuse treatment, the USA outstrips all other countries.

Unplanned de-institutionalization
Before adequate community care and housing was established, de-institutionalization was already underway.

Lack of long-term care provisions or planning
A lack of long-term care provision hampers progress.

Managed care and regulated review
In Europe this is familiar to planners looking for ways in which to cut costs.

Lack of a social welfare orientation
President Francois Mitterand in part attributed the Los Angeles riots to the lack of a social welfare orientation, to George Bush's great consternation (but with some truth).

Services research
During a 15-year period much work has been completed, including Stein and Test, the Robert Wood Johnson Foundation 9-Cities Program, the Inn at the Mass Mental Health Center, and the Institute of Medicine proposal on long-term care of vulnerable populations.

Quality control and outcome measures

University–public hospital linkage (Talbott and Robinowitz, 1986)

Research capacity
This includes basic science to treatment outcome research (Talbott, 1989).

Wealth
Differences in wealth are less given the strength of Western European economies, and due to finances, squandered in the USA on an inefficient care system (which does not provide adequate care for the poor, minorities and single-mother families).

Future steps

West–East

Information
Existing data, service descriptions, journals and books are essential; Central European countries are emerging from 50 years of isolation, as if they had been in a cave.

Money

Technical support
With planning efforts and programme design, more technical support is required. Visotsky has made a proposal for a mental health services resource similar to that in the USA's cooperative Agricultural Extension

Program. Such a repository of information about existing services, programme and research would be greatly welcomed (Visotsky, personal communication, 1978).

Sharing of problems not just solutions

As Bachrach (1988) has pointed out, experts on site must allow local situations to dictate programme provision, rather than grafting on 'model programmes' that are successful elsewhere. Too often, successes are presented, rather than our failures, while failures may be more instructive for those people planning de-institutionalization.

Research collaboration

THE WEST

Improvement in patient care should continue in the absence of definitive treatments or cures for the severe mental disorders through:

Services research

One ideal example of this is from Holder *et al.* (1991). This recent study showed the inverse ratio between cost and effectiveness of alcohol treatment options.

Basic research

Service provision before further de-institutionalization

ALL NATIONS

All countries can collaborate on research and service provision, of the types already pioneered by the US/UK Schizophrenia Project, developed by the WHO and promoted by the EC Committee on Mental Health and the countries of Central Europe, through their willingness to encourage different solutions. The Slovak Republic's plan for different regions to work out different solutions in their moves from asylum toward a balanced community care system, coupled with the West's financial and research help, could bring to light interesting naturalistic experiments in service provision (Ministry of Health, 1991).

Conclusion

When the problem of care of the severely and chronically mentally disordered people is approached from an international perspective, there is so much to be cautious about. But the similarities in the problems, the data bases used, and the possible solutions far outweigh the differences, despite different heritages, histories, ethnicities, languages, economics and administrative systems. Working together is more than a trite phrase; it is a necessity at this point in history.

References

Bachrach, L. L. (1988) On exporting and importing model programs. *Hospital and Community Psychiatry*, **39**, 1257–1258.

Bennett, D. H., Freeman, H. L. (1991) *Community Psychiatry: the Principles*. New York: Churchill Livingstone.

Braudel, F. (1986) *The Identity of France: Volume One: History and Environment*. New York: Harper and Row.

Freeman, H., Henderson, J. (1991) *Evaluation of Comprehensive Care of the Mentally Ill: the Transition from Mental Hospital Care to Extramural Care of the Mentally Ill in European Community Countries*. London: Washington, DC: APPI.

Holder, H., Longabaugh, R., Miller, W. R., Rubonis, A. V. (1991) The cost effectiveness of alcoholism. *Journal of Studies on Alcohol*, **52**, 517–540.

Hurst, J. W. (1991) Reforming health care in seven European nations. *Health Affairs*, **10**(1), 7–21.

Ministry of Health (1991) *The Reform of Psychiatric Care*. Members of a group of experts of the Ministry of Health of the Slovak Republic, May.

Sim, A. (1991) Even better services: a psychiatric perspective. *British Medical Journal*, **302**, 1061–1063.

Talbott, J. A. (ed.) (1989) *Future Directions for Psychiatry*. Washington, DC: American Psychiatric Association.

Talbott, J. A., Robinowitz C. B. (eds) (1986) *Working Together: State–University Collaboration in Mental Health*. Washington, DC: American Psychiatric Press, Inc.

Wasylenki, D., Goering, P., Macnaughton, E. (1992) Planning mental health services: I. background and key issues. *Canadian Journal of Psychiatry*, **37**, 199–206.

Chapter 14

Producing irreversible change: the process of transforming an old-fashioned hospital into a modern treatment centre

Fanny Duckert

Background

In 1985 Rogaland A-Senter (RAS) was a traditional hospital treating alcohol abusers. It consisted of two separate inpatient wards; one for longer stays (up to six months), and one for shorter stays (six to eight weeks). Outpatient treatment was given only sporadically, as was family therapy. Patients were admitted from all over Norway, although the majority of the patients came from the county of Rogaland. The hospital was privately owned, but funded by the State.

In 1985 a new law was passed, changing the basis for treatment of substance abusers. Previously, the treatment for substance abusers was a responsibility of the State. The State fully paid the costs of treatment and the county administration was at liberty to send clients to any hospital anywhere in the country. Following the new law, all this was changed and full responsibility shifted to the counties. A certain amount of money was allocated by the central government to each county, along with the new legislation requiring the county to provide a satisfactory treatment service for the substance abusers in their local region. In consequence the county of Rogaland had to reorganize their service system for alcohol addicts, and a plan for how to achieve this was made. It was decided that RAS was to be the main centre of treatment for alcohol abusers in the region. Additionally, it was intended that RAS was to do research, develop new treatment methods and provide educational services. However, this necessitated a major reorganization of the existing hospital. The hospital was privately owned, but run with financing from the state. The county took over the financial responsibilities and made out a contract for future cooperation.

One well-documented problem in organizational development is resistance to change (Robbins, 1979; Harvey and Brown, 1992). If there was not some resistance to change, organizational behaviour would take on characteristics of chaotic randomness, but this resistance also may hinder adaptation and progress. Many organizational development programmes do not take resistance forces seriously enough. Therefore, the changes often are short-lived and limited in scope. After a period everything more or less returns to the old situation.

The challenge for RAS was to transform the traditional hospital into a modern service centre, meeting the local population's needs for treatment of alcohol-related problems. In the summer of 1986 a reorganization process was started that lasted for about three years. The first step was to hire a new director to head the transformation process.

The information seeking process

Much information was collected about the structure and functions of the organization, and the relationship between the organization and the rest of the world. This implied reading all relevant documents, and participating in meetings with various administrative authorities and cooperation agencies. However, perhaps of most importance was to acquire knowledge of the staff and the organization culture (Schein, 1985).

All employees were personally interviewed, including technical and managerial staff (about 40 persons), giving each of them three questions: (1) What are your present work tasks? (2) If you were free to choose, what work tasks would you prefer to do? (3) If there was a discrepancy between 1 and 2 – What are the obstacles hindering you in doing what you most want to do?

There were several purposes to these interviews, including getting to know all the employees, and acquiring information about the individual capacities of the staff members. In this way an overview was obtained of non-utilized resources and talents that could be developed in the future. It was important to learn who felt comfortable with their jobs, and who felt misplaced. Imagined obstacles could be both persons and practical matters; this gave relevant information about possible ongoing problems in the organization. Also, different professional groups were instructed to make out memoranda outlining their special competencies, and what kind of tasks their group would be especially qualified to handle.

Participation occurred in all the different meetings at RAS, observing the interactions and communication patterns between the participants. Office doors were open, inviting people to enter if they had anything on their mind they wanted to share.

Problematic elements in the old organization

The established organizational structure was inspired by traditional therapeutic communities (Jones, 1953). The official organization structure was non-hierarchical and democratic, with little differences in tasks between the various professional groups.

Much energy was used on the daily running of the institution, leaving limited resources for the therapeutic work. The staff used considerable time and effort on inter-group conflicts and intrigues. Even if the ideal was one of equality and sharing of tasks, some tasks were more prestigious than others (e.g. doing individual therapy in a secluded office). There were a lot of complaints regarding heavy workloads; reciprocal accusations were more common between the different groups, about the others not taking their share of the workload.

There were few formal leaders, but a considerable number of quite powerful informal leaders. The lines of communication and decision-making were unclear and unstructured. Everywhere everyone was discussing all kinds of problems and exchanging informal information, but in formal meetings little of this was brought forward. Based upon which problems appeared during a meeting, all kind of decisions were taken in any kind of meeting. Much time was spent on long discussions, often with few conclusions. Decisions were made *ad hoc*, often based on superficial discussions, following the lead of the informal leaders. Shortly after, new problems often appeared, caused by unforeseen consequences following the last decision, leading to new superficial decisions, and so on.

Admission procedures were rigid. The clients had to be detoxified before admission. In the short-term ward, patients were admitted groupwise, once every three weeks, and participated in the same groups throughout the stay. However, due to drop-out, the groups were often significantly reduced before the end of treatment. In the long-term ward, new clients were admitted once a week, stayed for a longer period, and were more individually treated during the stay.

The long-term clients were generally older, more often homeless and unemployed, and more socially isolated than the short-term clients. Usually they had been referred to the clinic by social welfare agencies in order to dislodge them from their local environment. An organized plan for rehabilitation was rarely presented. The local agencies usually viewed the stay at the clinic as a resting period, both for the client in question, and for the milieu involved.

The short-term clients were somewhat more socially stable, and often had been referred by relatives or employers. But also for these clients, the stay was regularly considered as a time-out period for weary relatives, with scant involvement of people outside RAS.

The staff of RAS were usually left with the total responsibility of the clients, and had to handle all kinds of needs and problems. Cooperation problems with outside agencies were frequent. The staff complained about outsiders' ignorance, and that the clinic was looked upon as a 'garbage bin' into which problematic drunkards could be dumped.

From the cooperation agencies there were frequent complaints about low availability of services, short opening hours, and about rigid rules for admission. The clinic was also criticized for demanding sobriety before admittance. The lack of emergency services was often voiced.

Generally the clinic had a poor reputation, and was not an attractive working place for highly-skilled professionals. The wages were quite low, and few possibilities for career development existed within the organization. As a consequence, the employees generally were young and newly educated, staying only a short period before moving on to more attractive jobs, or they were persons with little formal education. It was problematic to get sufficient skilled applicants for vacant positions, and the absenteeism and turn-over rate were high among the employees.

Positive elements

The location and standards of the buildings were satisfactory. An interesting plan for the organization of treatment services for substance abusers in the county had just been proposed by the local authorities. In this plan Rogaland A-Senter had been given important tasks and responsibilities, and economic resources for handling these tasks had been promised.

The staff welcomed the possibility of a change. There had been considerable frustration among the employees because of the old organization. Several attempts at making changes had been done previously with variable success. The staff had expressed positive expectancies to the arrival on the scene of the new director.

Goals of the reorganization process

The theoretical background used was social learning theory (Bandura, 1977), and cognitive/behaviourial therapy (Liberman *et al.*, 1975; Beck, 1976). In this model, substance abuse is looked upon as learned behaviour and as a life-style problem (Pattison *et al.*, 1977; Miller and Mastria, 1977; Duckert, 1981). The destructive drinking pattern is developed, and maintained through reciprocal reinforcement between the individual and his or her milieu. The problem involves relatives, friends and colleagues. It is important to reach problem drinkers as soon as possible, prior to the problems becoming too serious. In order to change the problem drinking, the relationships and interaction processes must be addressed in the therapy. Also the families of problem drinkers need proper assistance.

As an implication of the above notions, the development of early intervention programmes was seen as necessary. Outpatient treatment should be the rule, involving the family and relevant network. Treatment should be non-stigmatic, flexible, and easily available. Inpatient treatment periods should be as short as possible, and mainly be reserved for emergency situations.

The main goals of the reorganization were:

- Increase the capacity and quality of treatment
- Establish new treatment services
- Make treatment services more easily available
- Attract new groups of clients
- Establish research and educational activities
- Improve the reputation of the organization, making it a more respected cooperation partner for the outside world, and a more attractive workplace for highly skilled professionals
- Decrease turnover and absenteeism among the employees.

The change process

The change process mainly took place over a period of three years.

The period of planning and preparation

A working group was established, consisting of the director, the administrative manager, the heads of the two departments (both psychologists), and one representative for each of the two other main professions – social workers and nurses. The planning group met one day per week during a period of four months, in order to develop the new organizational plan. This work was based on the county's plan, the staff's written and oral descriptions and wishes for future tasks, in addition to the new ideas about the organization.

The various groups the institution wanted to reach with its services were identified. Three main target groups were recognized: (a) early problem drinkers; (b) hidden, but socially stable problem drinkers: (c) serious problem drinkers, with additional social problems. Within all these groups, sex and age would lead to further differentiation. Thereafter the treatment needs of each of the identified groups were outlined. What kind of therapeutic assistance would they require, and how should the institution be designed to meet these needs? The new organization plan for the institution gradually appeared.

Treatment services were to be centred in the new outpatient unit, which would be staffed with highly skilled professionals. All referrals were to be taken care of by the admission team, who also made the initial assessment of the referred client. In most cases the outpatient unit also would be responsible for the further treatment. In the case of a client having children under the age of thirteen, the person was to be referred to the family treatment unit, who would be responsible for further treatment. Also the family treatment unit would mainly work with outpatient treatment, but, in addition, they would have at their disposal three flats, which could be used if inpatient treatment turned out to be necessary.

As part of the family unit services, a nursery school was to be established, aimed at the children involved in treatment. The nursery school was to be staffed for observation and for giving parental guidance to the adults. The stable group of children was to be the children of the staff, while the children of the clients would spend variable periods of time in the nursery school.

The admission team could also refer patients for treatment in the inpatient unit. This unit was to have a section for emergency admissions, where clients could be admitted for immediate care, either because of intoxication or other immediate crises. After the emergency phase, the client was either to go on with outpatient treatment or to go through a four weeks' inpatient treatment programme. In addition to the above units an educational and research unit was to be establishead.

After the design of the institution was fulfilled, the staffing of each unit was decided. Detailed job descriptions for all positions were made. The new organization plan and the job descriptions were handed out to all staff members through their workers' union representatives, and each professional group was asked to give their written comments. These were then worked into the revised organization plan. The final plan was presented to the board of the institution for discussion and approval. Thereafter the new organization plan was forwarded to county authorities for final approval. This process lasted about six months.

The year of transition

In preparation for the reorganization, the long-term inpatient ward had been closed down and rebuilt to accommodate the outpatient unit, the family unit, and the educational/research unit. The short-time inpatient unit had been renovated to accommodate the emergency ward. The administrative unit was to be moved into a new section. These preparations had been done during the last period of the planning process (when informal approval of the new plan by the local authorities had been received).

Parallel to the planning process there was also a series of information meetings and discussions with the employees. By the time the new organization plan was ready, and the job descriptions completed, all the employees were asked to indicate their preferences for future positions in the new organization. Based upon this, and their earlier written presentations, the employees were fitted into the new institution.

The major transition took place at the beginning of January 1986. The institution was completely closed down for one week. The entire staff went by bus to a hotel in the mountains, a couple of hours drive away. It had been underlined that everyone should participate in this process, including the technical and managerial staff. The next three days were intensive, with lectures, information, discussions, marathon group sessions, role playing, and enthusiasm-raising activities, in order to prepare everyone for the changes scheduled to take place.

This session ended on the evening of the third day, and the following two days were scheduled for moving. Everyone had been given a new office, and was to move during these two days. The furniture left over after the rebuilding was available for everyone to use in their new offices. When everyone had taken what they wanted, money for supplying additional needs, such as curtains and flowers, was granted. Thus everyone started the new year in their own, newly furnished office.

The employees were also to have new tasks and responsibilities. Most of the staff members wanted to do some kind of therapeutic work, and had beforehand stated their wishes for which kind of therapy activities they wanted to take part in. Based upon the available therapeutic resources, a group therapy programme for the inpatient unit was established. Each group was run by a professional therapist, together with one or two less experienced cotherapists. In this way the experienced leaders trained the less experienced.

All the professionals, including those in the outpatient units, were engaged in running groups in the inpatient unit. Thus the different units were more closely knitted together, and the inpatient unit could profit from the special expertise in the outpatient units. In this way the inpatient treatment was intensified. Many of the group activities were also available for outpatients. In addition, special outpatient groups were established (e.g. groups for relatives and control training for early problem drinkers).

To increase the availability and attractiveness of treatment services, several changes were made:

- The new emergency ward in the inpatient unit was staffed all day and night, and at weekends. The staff were authorized to admit patients outside normal opening hours. The client could remain in the emergency section for up to three days, giving the regular admittance team the possibility to make the necessary assessments for possible further treatment.
- The working hours of the treatment staff were adjusted. Once a week everyone had to work at night. This implied that instead of working from 8.00 until 15.30, on this day, he or she was scheduled to work from 12.00 until 19.30. A modest economical compensation was given for the off-scheduled hours. Each unit was responsible for covering every ordinary weekday but had freedom in deciding who should work late which day within the unit. With this adjustment, the institution could offer professional assistance until 19.30 on all weekdays.
- Contacts were made with local newspapers and the local radio

station, presenting the new treatment profile, and the new treatment possibilities the institution could offer. The ideological perspectives were presented, and the advantages of early intervention were underlined. The treatment opportunities for families, spouses and children were also advertised.

In cooperation with the local radio programme a series of six short programmes about alcohol problems and treatment were made and broadcast once a week. The goal of the programme was to demystify alcohol problems, to make them a topic for discussion and understanding, and to make help-seeking non-stigmatizing.

- A new, big car park was opened, and facilities for seminars and meetings were made available in one of the buildings. This made it possible to arrange seminars, courses and meetings on a regular basis. As a consequence there was a significant increase in the number of persons passing through the doors of the institution each day, many of whom were non-clients. The old stigma attached to visitors of the institution gradually disappeared, and made it easier for clients to visit without being noticed. This increased the possibility of recruiting new clients, who before had stayed away, fearing the stigma of being labelled as alcoholics.

  The new facilities also gave opportunities for inviting cooperation agencies to meetings and seminars. Many of the participants had not previously visited the institution and were pleasantly surprised by what they encountered. Gradually this enhanced the status of the centre.

- The cooperation problems with the outside world, which had resulted in professional isolation and lack of communication, were attended to. RAS had often been made use of by the rest of the health and social welfare system as a temporary place to get rid of burdensome and hopeless cases. After referring the client the referral agency usually had withdrawn all engagements, and hoped for RAS to keep the client away as long as possible. The staff of RAS were then left with all responsibilities, and in addition to the treatment often had to take care of practical and social problems, for instance, finding the client a job or a place to live. On the other hand, cooperation agencies often complained about the inflexible and bureaucratic procedures for admission to RAS and its unwillingness to give assistance in emergency situations.

After the reorganization, RAS services were greatly improved. Consequently, the centre gained a better position for making demands on cooperation agencies. One demand was that the referral agency should remain responsible for the client throughout the treatment stay. Definite plans for further arrangements after the end of stay should be made before seeking admittance to RAS. Without adequate plans for individual rehabilitation, admittance to RAS was not possible. On the other hand, when part of an adequate plan for the client, quick admittance was guaranteed. The services of the centre were also available during the follow-up procedure, and quick readmittance offered whenever necessary in acute phases of the rehabilitation programme.

First, several of the cooperation agencies protested against the new demands from RAS. However, discussion meetings were arranged, and information about the background of the changes was distributed. Soon the agencies also discovered that the services of RAS were greatly improved, and that the cooperation in each case went more smoothly.

Inducing irreversible changes

The major challenge during the reorganization process had been to make changes without the possibility of returning to the old system. Several strategies with the intention of producing irreversible changes were used:

- Making the staff committed during the process. Information was continuously given as part of the planning process. A close relationship with the employees' union was developed, thereby establishing them as the main channel of reciprocal information. The union delegates were continuously kept informed about the process, and were given responsibility for passing this information on to the members of their various unions. They were also responsible for bringing back the comments from their colleagues to the planning group. Criticism and suggestions had to be written down to ensure consideration.

  Another strategy for increasing commitment was to make each employee express his or her capacities and wishes for tasks and positions in the new organization. The presented wishes were accommodated as far as possible in the new organization plan. This was based on a strong belief that most people who can influence their own work situation and can do what they enjoy, do a better job. This will also increase commitment to the workplace (Luthans, 1992).

- Breaking up old affiliations. In the old system there were many informal affiliations among the employees based upon both geographical and working closeness. Many of the employees knew few persons outside these close alliances. Such structures could easily become obstacles to the planned organizational development. Much of the group work carried out during the first seminar preceding the reorganization introduced the employees to colleagues that they previously had made little contact with, thus making the whole staff more familiar with each other. The reorganization of all units and the reallocation of all staff members into new offices were an essential part of making the changes irreversible. From then on it would be impossible to revert to the old system and the old alliances.

- Diminishing the possibilities for informal leadership. In the new organization more unambiguous channels for communication and decision making were established. The above mentioned strategies for making employees more committed to the new organization, and the breaking up of old alliances, reduced the possibility for 'shadow cabinets' to appear in the new organization. An alternative system for advancement in the organization was developed, based on a combination of formal education, personal skills and time in the system. Several of the positions were adjusted upwards, both regarding titles and salaries, and new leading positions were established. Some of the old informal leaders were offered possibilities to increase their formal qualifications, enabling them to compete for more formal positions.

- 'Learning by doing.' One resistance to change is the individual fear of trying something new. This is often demonstrated by an endless demand for preparations before starting up new activities. The principle of 'learning by doing' was therefore established. After an introduction and a short period of preparation, all staff members were 'thrown into' new tasks rather quickly. All the new groups started at the same time. The first period was defined as a period of trial and error, with a summing up of the experiences after six and twelve months. During these periods several evaluation meetings were held, each summing up experiences and adjusting the contents and structure of the groups.

- 'Acting as if.' Another important part of the change process was to use the employees as 'ambassadors' to the rest of the world. Previously, work morale and loyalty towards the institution among the employees had been rather low. It was common for the employees to complain about their working place. In the new system all the employees were asked if they wanted to have information tasks. The majority answered yes to this. All kinds of relevant social activities to which the employees participated, for instance charity groups, parent groups, youth groups, various sports groups, religious groups, social groups, and so on, were registered. Before entering the information tasks, the educational department furnished the employees with necessary information material and offered training in presentation techniques. Also the employees were allowed a compensation for the work they put into information tasks.

  One of the consequences of this approach was that the employees started to voice a much more enthusiastic attitude towards their working place, not only when on an official mission, but also privately, and when on the job. This change is in accordance with previous knowledge that role-playing of attitude positions can strongly influence the personal attitudes of the role-players (Zimbardo and Ebbesen, 1970).

- Lobbying. In the end the new organization plan had to be approved by the county administration and the local politicians. It was important to receive acceptance of the whole plan, and not open up possibilities for cutting back on any of the planned activities, reducing the chance of lasting change.

  Intensive lobbying was therefore necessary. Among the employees, several were politically active within a wide variety of political parties, and could be used as sources of influence to their political allies in the elected county political groups. The strategy was to contact the various political parties, informing the representatives of the new plan, pointing out the elements that would be of special interest to that political group. In this way support from enough politicians to obtain acceptance of the new organization plan was secured.

The year of consolidation

The second year of change also started with a three-day seminar for the entire staff at a hotel in the mountains. This time the main task was to analyse the experience gained in the first year. The staff were responsible for reporting from the different units, and the professional activities. Problems and successes were registered.

For the second year some adjustments in the treatment programme were made, the educational programme was expanded, and research activities were started. Further organizational development was also made. In cooperation with the Unit for Social Sciences and Communication at the local college, the heads of the units started up a leadership training programme, allocating one day a week for one year.

Challenges to be met during this period were:

- Since more and more treatment was done on an outpatient basis, the remaining inpatients became more selected and had more serious problems. Also the emergency ward received clients who were in a more desperate situation than previously experienced at the centre. This implied that inpatient treatment became more demanding and heavy for the staff.
- The organization often experienced intergroup conflicts between the different units, and it was sometimes difficult to make employees in one unit undertake tasks in another unit. For instance, the staff from the family unit or the outpatient unit were not always eager to fulfil their group therapy responsibilities in the inpatient unit.
- Also if the staff from other units wanted a stay in the inpatient unit for their clients, conflicts often arose about whom should be the main responsible therapist for the client during the stay.
- Even if most of the staff members expressed wishes for doing more therapeutic work, not all ended up by feeling comfortable with such tasks.

   In the old system such problems would have been floating around, not openly discussed, but creating much distress and frustration. In the new organization it was underlined that problems and negative experiences should be brought into the open, and be handled in a constructive way. With more clear and unambiguous channels for information and decisions it was easier to know where and how to present problems. As a rule, the person or the group that gave expression to a certain problem, also was expected to give suggestions for solving the problem in question.
Once every six months an evaluation of the treatment structure was

done, and adjustments made. In preparation for this, the staff members were asked to indicate which preferences they had for the next period, as to treatment and administrative tasks. Within reason they were given the possibility to switch between tasks. Thus, they could try out different jobs, and after a period decide whether they wanted to go on with that task, return to old ones, or try another task. This modified version of job-rotation made the system flexible with a lot of possibilities for personal development. Of course, the wishes presented had to be adjusted, so that the total number of tasks was adhered to.

Less attractive tasks, as for instance serving in the emergency ward, were covered by a system of 6 months' engagements. Thus the staff members could try out the tasks for a limited period of time, and if they did not feel comfortable they could change tasks after that. After a while it often turned out that some of the employees liked that kind of work, and therefore chose to keep on with the tasks. In the case of the emergency ward, the nurses in particular became the stable staff members. Thus, after the initial period, the emergency ward did not constitute a staffing problem.

The period of departure

It was important that the process of change should not be halted by management changes. The final six months were focused on making the organization less dependent on one specific leader. The director's personal involvement in the organization was gradually withdrawn.

During the previous year the heads of the units had graduated from the leadership development programme, and more independence could be given to each of them. Decisions concerning only one unit could be taken by the head of that unit. Decisions inflicting consequences on other units should be taken by the board of the units' heads, together with the director and administrative head.

The last couple of months were mainly used for introducing the new director to the system and going through the appropriate 'rites de passages' with the institution.

Results

Despite tremendous organizational changes, the number of persons treated at the institution did not decrease during the period of transition. There was an increase in the number of self-referrals and the number of persons with no previous treatment also increased. The ratio of women increased from about 10% to 30% (Table 14.1).

Table 14.1 Treatment activity per year

	1985	1986	1987	1988
The number of inpatient admissions	273	235	409	573
Number of inpatient days	10 930	7636	5961	5945
Number of outpatient consultations	0	1103	3136	3298
Number of families	0	0	24	50

In 1990, Rogaland A-Senter received an award by the Ministry of Health and Social Affairs, and the Association of County Authorities, acclaiming RAS' successful reorganization and outstanding service to members of the community in need of help for alcohol-related problems.

A series of cooperation projects with other health and social agencies was established, and educational activities (e.g. seminars, courses, discussion groups), were frequent.

The turnover and absenteeism among the employees were significantly reduced during this period. RAS became a more attractive place to work, which for instance was registered in the increasing number of well-qualified applicants for new and vacant positions.

Thus, most of the intended changes had been carried through as planned.

In 1996, RAS was appointed as one of the seven national centres of competency, with special responsibility for addressing the questions related to alcohol-related problems in the workplace.

Implications

Treatment services for persons with alcohol problems in Norway had traditionally, as in many other western countries, been aimed at 'alcoholics' – long-term problem drinkers who belong to the lower strata of society. Less concern had been devoted to the socially well-adapted problem drinkers in the early stages of drinking. The contents of treatment had been deeply tainted by perceptions of the unmotivated, unaware and dissimulating alcoholic who must forcibly be persuaded in various ways to accept treatment. Treatment had largely involved confronting the problem drinker with the adverse consequences of his or her present life style, pressuring him or her to 'acknowledge' the 'alcoholism' [sic] and the subsequent need to engage in total abstinence for the rest of his or her life.

The reorganization of Rogaland A-Senter was based on the awareness that an increase in alcohol consumption is the decisive factor behind a number of the most serious accidents and injuries, and that drinking increases a number of problems directly or indirectly related to alcohol. Another important factor was the realization of problem drinking as a complex, multifaceted phenomenon which does not only involve the individual, but also the environment, and the observation that problems vary not only from person to person, but from one period to another, or one situation to another for the same person. A person's drinking pattern is strongly influenced by the prevailing social environment. Subsequently the traditional dividing lines between the various stages of alcoholism has faded, for example the magic dividing line between abuse and irreversible alcoholism (Duckert, 1993).

The flaws in the traditional approaches to treatment have become more apparent as attitudes have changed toward alcohol-related problems. Generally, increasing emphasis is now placed on outpatient treatment within the problem drinker's immediate environment, and on a broadening cooperation between specialists and the general health and social service sector. Primary health care is also showing growing concern over the effect of alcohol on diseases with other diagnoses, and recognizes the need for altering the drinking pattern of a large number of patients to improve the results. Furthermore, a shift in emphasis from institutional treatment to various forms of early intervention and minimum treatment is notable (US Institute of Medicine, 1990).

By using relatively simple measures, alcohol consumption can be reduced with subsequent favourable effects on the general health status. Large groups of problem drinkers can be reached through the general health sector at reasonable costs, without recourse to costly specialized institutions.

The process of change described above is one example of how to conduct a reorganization aimed at transforming an old-fashioned 'alcoholism' treatment hospital into a modern treatment centre for persons with alcohol-related problems. During the transformation, many of the old fences between substance abuse treatment and the other health and social welfare agencies were removed. But still there is more to be done. The ultimate goal must be to integrate the public responsibility for secondary prevention and treatment as fully as possible into the ordinary services for health and social care.

References

Bandura, A. (1977) *Social Learning Theory*. Englewood Cliffs, NJ: Prentice Hall.

Beck, A. (1976) *Cognitive Therapy and the Emotional Disorders*. New York: Meridan, New American Library.

Duckert, F. (1981) Behavioral analysis of the drinking pattern of alcoholics – with special focus on degree of control in different situations. *Scandinavian Journal of Behavioral Therapy*, **10**, 121–133.

Duckert, F. (1993) Alcohol problems and treatment: follow up studies of problem drinkers with special reference to drinking behaviour. Doctoral dissertation, National Institute for Alcohol and Drug Research, Oslo.

Harvey, D. F., Brown, D. R (1992) *An Experimental Approach to Organization Development*. London: Prentice-Hall International Editions.

Jones, M. (1953) *The Therapeutic Community: A New Treatment Method in Psychiatry*. New York: Basic Books.

Liberman, R. P., King, L. W., DeRisi, W. J., McCann, M. (1975) *Personal Effectiveness – Guiding People to Assert Themselves and Improve Their Social Skills*. Champaign: Research Press.

Luthans, F. (1992) *Organizational Behavior*. Singapore: McGraw-Hill.

Miller, P. M., Mastria, M. A. (1977) *Alternatives to Alcohol Abuse – a Social Learning Model*. Champaign: Research Press.

Pattison, E. M., Sobell, M. B., Sobell, L. C. (1977) *Emerging Concepts of Alcohol Dependence*. New York: Springer Publishing Company.

Robbins, S. P. (1979) *Organizational Behavior – Concepts, Controversies, and Applications*. London: Prentice-Hall International Editions.

Schein, E. (1985) *Organizational Culture and Leadership. A Dynamic View*. New York: Jossey-Bass Inc.

US Institute of Medicine (1990) *Broadening the Base of Treatment for Alcohol Problems*. Washington: National Academy Press.

Zimbardo, P., Ebbesen, E. B. (1970) *Influencing Attitudes and Changing Behavior*. Reading, Mass: Addison-Wesley Publishing Company.

Chapter 15

Survivor-led research in human services: challenging the dominant medical paradigm

Jan Wallcraft

The problem with orthodox mental health research

Scientific research, as many twentieth century philosophers and sociologists of science have been at pains to point out, is not just a matter of neutral observation and recording of natural and self-evident facts. Scientific training imposes a set of interpretations, categories and meanings on to the scientists' sense impressions. Scientific means for collecting information, whether this relies mainly on technological equipment such as the microscope, or techniques of information-gathering such as the intelligence test, work within a paradigm, or world-view. The methods of discovery have built into them assumptions about the meaning and relevance of the facts they reveal. Facts do not speak for themselves. Scientific method is a creative, human fallible process, culturally determined and akin to other cultural artefacts such as literature, art and magic.

Natural scientists have to learn to see cells through a microscope and social scientists have to be taught the significance of a sociological survey. This learning is conditioned by the prevailing normal science paradigm – both the overarching paradigm of western scientific method, with its legacy of logical positivist deduction, Cartesian dualism, Newtonian two-variable reductionism, Popperian logical falsification, and the paradigms which govern each separate scientific discipline. Each branch of science has its own history, its legendary pioneers and its body of accepted facts, theories and methodologies. Just as the development of the microscope resulted from a belief that all nature could be explained by examining the minute building blocks from which it was formed, so psychiatric diagnostic methods, such as the DSM IV and depression rating scales were developed out of a belief that the human psyche could be understood if it were submitted to a close, clinical and objective scrutiny by neutral and highly trained scientists.

Western mental health research is a product of a western culture which has embedded within it a history of imperialism, xenophobia, male supremacy, and class division. The dominant group delimited the scope of rationality to that which was reasonable, acceptable and comprehensible to itself, and then based its sciences on this narrow area of rationality, regarding the belief systems of others as worthy of investigation, but treating its own belief system as self-evidently true.

Medical science, and psychiatry in particular, have adopted a positivist and reductionist paradigm which has distanced their practitioners from the subjects of their intervention and dehumanized both professional and patient. Psychiatric research emanating from such a world-view, or paradigm, inevitably negates the truths of the majority of those who come within its scope, and is therefore likely to be experienced as disempowering, oppressive and damaging if viewed from the perspective of most of its recipients. Mental health research from a service user, or psychiatric survivor perspective, is beginning to reveal the truth of these statements, and to show the need for a new paradigm in mental health research.

Kuhn (1970) argues that 'normal science is predicated on the assumption that the scientific community knows what the world is like', and 'is a strenuous and devoted attempt to force nature into the conceptual boxes supplied by the paradigm'. Paradigms are not abandoned simply because mismatches are found between the paradigm and reality – these are generally seen as problems to be resolved by further exploration. However, if normal science persistently fails to find satisfactory answers to the problems of its day, the paradigm may go into a crisis, and scientists will begin casting about for new ways to frame their enquiries, new methods, new conceptualizations. The transition from one paradigm to another cannot be made, Kuhn says, one step at a time, but is more like a conversion experience, or a gestalt switch to a new way of seeing.

In medicine, technologies and techniques of data-gathering developed since the nineteenth century have been dogged by criticism on the grounds that they have increasingly distanced physicians from their patients, and that the technique or technology used shapes the physician's view of the patient's disease pattern.

The technique chosen does more than generate a particular kind of fact – it influences human attitudes and relationships. Techniques influence the relationship of the patient with the physician; they influence the doctor's image of himself/herself as a decision-maker; they influence the association of physicians with each other, and thus the manner in which the institutions of medical practice are organized. Attitudinal and relational changes such as these are often not recognized, but they are crucial, and physicians should consider them in evaluating the benefits and harm of different fact-gathering techniques (Reiser, 1978).

New paradigms in physics, from Einstein's theory of relativity to Capra's discussion of quantum interconnectedness (Capra, 1983) and its relation to eastern mysticism have as yet scarcely touched mainstream medical theory, which still highly values the quest for scientific neutrality, objectivity and empirical positivism.

Mental health research, from its earliest origins, has chosen to ignore the views of the recipients of diagnosis and treatment. This is typified by the horrifyingly cold, inhumane (but superficially objective) tone in which an eighteenth century physician details his experiments with pouring cold water over the head of a woman whose main symptom was an unwillingness to sleep with her husband. The volume and frequency of the applications of cold water poured on her head are monitored, and the successful result – a docile and willing woman returned to her marital duty – faithfully recorded. As Blair (1982) comments, the amount and force of the water discharged on patients' heads was measurable and so could be calculated, which gave it a scientific flavour. The dose was determined according to the tenacity with which the mad person clung to his or her delusional feeling … or refused to be normalized.

Here is a prototype for modern psychiatric research on treatments such as ECT and medication. Clinical trials of ECT measure only what is accessible to objective measurement, such as the voltage used and the frequency of treatments. The patient's subjective experience is transformed into quantitative measures of observed behaviour or omitted as unmeasurable and therefore irrelevant. Anecdotally, doctors tend to report successful treatment in normative terms. They boast of returning the patient to the bosom of her or his family, apparently cured of the pathology of not behaving in the ways others expected of them. The subsequent quality of the former patient's life, or the frequency of their re-hospitalization has rarely been a subject of clinical interest.

When mental patients' opinions are canvassed, until recently this was almost always done within a medical framework. The researchers tended to be clinicians – psychiatrists, psychologists, medical students and occasionally nursing students, already well on the way to being socialized into the normal science paradigm for their particular field of expertise.

Voluntary organizations, such as MIND, though concerned with combating the stigma of mental illness and improving treatment and patients' rights, were, until the late 1980s, very strongly influenced by psychiatrists. These organizations rarely challenged their diagnostic procedures or the objective reality of psychiatric illness categories. Because of the status of normal science and the dominance of medicine in psychiatry, most research funding and academic credibility attaches to research done within the medical paradigm. Research done by voluntary organizations, therefore, was generally careful to avoid directly challenging medical knowledge or encroaching on areas which had been claimed as the field of the clinicians. This is not to deny the existence of a dissident stream of research and writing which countered the positivistic claims of psychiatry. Much of this was done, however, by psychiatrists, clinical psychologists and neurologists, who had sufficient scientific credibility to challenge the power of the orthodox paradigm.

Though the work of radical psychiatrists such as Laing (1970), Szasz (1974), Cooper (1978) and Breggin (1993) has been influential and important for many mental health workers and patients, they have often suffered for their rebellion, being marginalized as oddballs and mavericks by their colleagues. Their work has not had a major impact on psychiatric practice, despite claims to a more eclectic approach in modern psychiatric textbooks (e.g. Sims and Owens, 1993). Funding, legal status and credibility have remained with the practitioners of normal science in psychiatry, and other organizations wanting to work in the field of mental health, including social workers and voluntary organizations have, until recently, had to accept the dominance of the medical model. From the nineteenth century onwards, most major fields of study of the human psyche have laid claim to scientific credentials. Even Freud strove to frame his concept of functional disorders in similar terms to physical disorders, and believed that eventually neurological and biochemical explanations of neurosis would be forthcoming.

Psychiatrists have spent much of the past 150 years conducting ruthlessly clinical and inhumane experiments on unwilling, uninformed or poorly-informed subjects – testing on them treatments ranging from physical restraint and induced hypothermia through a variety of means of inducing shock and convulsions and the effects of different ways of applying electricity, through a vast range of toxic chemicals to behaviour modification regimens. This experimentation still continues. For instance, despite the fact that new psychotropic drugs such as Prozac and clozapine are already associated with some serious adverse effects, they are currently being promoted as safe and effective remedies for depression and schizophrenia respectively.

The prospective recipients of these treatments have not been consulted about any aspect of the experimentation; neither the legitimacy of the treatment goals, the method of ascertaining successful results or the weighting of cost-benefit considerations of possible iatrogenic effects of treatment. People are rarely privy to full information about their treatments or the risks they are being expected to take as guinea pigs for the latest experiment in behaviour control. When they experience the adverse effects, their point of view is usually either ignored, or treated as deeply suspect, on the grounds that mental patients do not know what is best for them and may be imagining or exaggerating their problems. Complaints about treatment have frequently been dismissed as further symptoms of illness.

Psychiatry has not been through a Kuhnian scientific revolution – its paradigm has not changed in the past 200 years. Psychiatrists have disowned none of the knowledge gleaned through inhumane experimentation on a captive population – proceeding instead in very gradual, incremental steps. Many of these steps contribute more to putting a new gloss on empirically-based psychiatric beliefs such as the therapeutic benefits of induced shock and sedation. One can be justified in asking, what kind of knowledge can be established by such means? Does psychiatric research provide an understanding of how to help troubled people, or an increasingly efficient technology of social oppression? In what way has free world psychiatric experimentation and treatment differed from that carried out by Soviet or Nazi psychiatrists?

Meanwhile, at the leading edge of hard science, physicists have long since learned the limits of objectivity, and begun to recognize the observer effect (Capra, 1983; Prigogine and Stengers, 1984). Imposing categories on nature forces nature to confirm our beliefs. Questionnaires designed and administered by clinicians elicit only the information they are designed to elicit, which tends to reinforce the belief system of those who designed it. Such information, determined by a hegemonic belief system, and constantly reinforced by it, can only be a partial reflection of an infinitely complex reality.

In western science, the dominant rationalist Cartesian world-view underpinning science blinded it to the day-to-day realities, cultures and beliefs of the majority of the population. Mainstream human sciences have been slow to address the lived experience of black people, women, working-class people, Asian people, disabled people, lesbian or gay people, people outside the 18–65 age range, and even many of the people who are apparently its main beneficiaries – upper and middle class white males.

But the proliferation, in the second half of the twentieth century, of critiques from inside and outside the scientific establishment, give indications that the Age of Reason, of positivism and certainty in the dominant science and culture, has had its heyday and is now in decline. Momentum is building for a Kuhnian paradigm shift in western scientific thinking, in both human and physical sciences. A new paradigm will bring in new models and new methods of seeking knowledge.

Positivism in science is gradually being replaced by realist or existentialist science. Realism in science is described by Rom Harre (1981):

> Most realists would argue that facts and theories are not independent. Facts are revealed to a human observer who uses a theory to identify significant items from the complex flux of experience. It follows that a realist can admit that there may be real indeterminateness in the world.

The realist does not deny the existence of objective reality, but regards it as infinitely complex and unpredictable. An observer cannot see and describe aspects of reality without a set of prior metaphysical assumptions, which should be made open to the scrutiny of others along with the facts selected and conclusions drawn.

Existentialism in science is described by the systems theorist Schon (1971) in the following terms:

> In existentialism, it is taken as given that situations of public action contain more information than we can handle and are inherently unstable. Within them, then, knowledge can have only the validity it is found to have in the here-and-now. The here-and-now provides the test, the source, and the limit of knowledge. No theory drawn from past

experience may be taken as literally applicable to this situation, nor will a theory based on the experience of this situation prove literally applicable to the next situation.

According to Harre and Schon, theories (and the facts which flow from them), are human creative constructs, not discoveries of objective reality, and are only as good as the results they achieve in the here-and-now. If people on the receiving end of psychiatric services are not satisfied with the services and disagree with the philosophical model in which these services reside, then psychiatric theory and its underpinning assumptions need revision.

All mental health research which treats distressed people, patients or clients as the object of clinical study, devaluing their lived reality and subjecting the totality of their experience to a reductionist, atomistic, impersonal set of diagnostic tests must lead to incomplete and misleading results. A service built on a scientific paradigm which submits lived experience to a medical model dominated by biochemical and genetic theories of mental illness is inevitably dehumanizing and disempowering – for both recipients and providers. Treatments based on a limited and partial understanding of the patient's reality deny many aspects of the whole human being and devalue his or her perceptions, thus denying the patient's power to define and heal herself/himself and often creating long-term dependency on experts and institutional care. Incremental reforms will never be sufficient. What is needed is nothing less than a scientific revolution in psychiatry. A user perspective cannot be held valid at the same time as a medical perspective – they are, generally speaking, incompatible world-views.

This is a wide-ranging, and maybe controversial claim, but it is borne out by the evidence of almost every study that has been done which has genuinely offered current and former mental patients the opportunity to state their views in their own words, without the imposition of a medical framework.

Mental health services based on scientific research have, for the past 150 years at least, been consistently criticized by a substantial minority of their recipients. One of the earliest accounts is that of John Perceval in the 1830s. Perceval, the son of the assassinated Prime Minister, was confined to two different private madhouses in 1831–1834. In 1835 he began writing about his experiences as a patient. He describes his visions and delusions, and what they caused him to do, then goes on to describe the oppressiveness of his treatment. These descriptions are remarkably similar to those frequently heard in the literature of the current mental health self-advocacy movement:

> Now with regard to my treatment, I have to make at first two general observations, which apply, I am afraid, too extensively to every system of management yet employed towards persons in my condition.
>
> First, the suspicion and the fact of my being incapable of reasoning correctly, or deranged in understanding, justified apparently every person who came near me, in dealing with me also in a manner contrary to reason and contrary to nature...
>
> Secondly, my being likely to attack the rights of others gave these individual licence, in every respect, to trample upon mine... Instead of my understanding being addressed and enlightened, and of my path being made as clear and plain as possible, in consideration of my confusion, I was committed, in really difficult and mysterious circumstances, calculated of themselves to confound my mind, even if in a sane state, to unknown and untried hands; and I was placed amongst strangers, without introduction, explanation or exhortation (Peterson, 1982).

Rae Unzicker, coordinator of the National Association of Psychiatric Survivors in the USA described the twentieth century position of a mental patient in the following poem:

> To be a mental patient is to be stigmatized, ostracized, socialized, patronized, psychiatrized.
>
> To be a mental patient is to have everyone controlling your life but you. You're watched by your shrink, your social worker, your friends, your family. And then you're diagnosed as paranoid.
>
> To be a mental patient is to live with the constant threat and possibility of being locked up at any time, for almost any reason.
>
> To be a mental patient is to live on $82 a month in food stamps, which won't let you buy the Kleenex to dry your tears. And to watch your shrink come back to his office from lunch, driving a Mercedes Benz.
>
> To be a mental patient is to take drugs that dull your mind, leaden your senses, make you jitter and drool, and then you take more drugs to lessen the side effects.
>
> To be a mental patient is to apply for jobs and lie about how you've spent the last few months or years, because you've been in the hospital, and then you don't get the job anyway, because you're a mental patient.
>
> To be a mental patient is to watch TV and see shows about how violent and dangerous and dumb and incompetent and crazy you are.
>
> To be a mental patient is not to matter.

To be a mental patient is never to be taken seriously.

To be a mental patient is to be a resident of a ghetto, surrounded by other mental patients who are as scared and hungry and bored and broke as you are.

To be a mental patient is to be a statistic.

To be a mental patient is to wear a label, a label that never goes away, a label that says little about what you are and even less about who you are.

To be a mental patient is never to say what you mean, but to sound like you mean what you say.

To be a mental patient is to tell your psychiatrist he's helping you, even if he's not.

To be a mental patient is to act glad when you're sad and calm when you're mad and to always be appropriate.

To be a mental patient is to participate in stupid groups that call themselves therapy. Music isn't music, it's therapy; volleyball isn't a sport, it's therapy; sewing is therapy; washing dishes is therapy. Even the air you breathe is therapy, and that's called the milieu.

To be a mental patient is not to die, even if you want to – and not cry, and not hurt, and not be scared, and not be angry, and not be vulnerable, and not laugh too loud

– because if you do you only prove you are a mental patient
even if you are not.

And so you become a no-thing in a no-world, and you are not.
(Unzicker, 1984).

Autobiographical accounts and poetry can give us an insight into how psychiatry is experienced which is completely absent from most clinical psychiatric research. Mental health research must find ways to include the stories of the recipients of psychiatry, told in their own words.

Towards research methods to create a new paradigm in mental health

Reason and Rowan (1981) list a number of general criticisms of scientific orthodoxy in research. All are extremely pertinent to why traditional mental health research supports and perpetuates oppressive treatments and services.

A few of these are summarized below:

- Model of the person – people are seen as isolable from their normal social contexts.

- Reductionism – studying variables, rather than persons or groups, is a flight from knowing people and groups as wholes.
- Deception – lying, arrogance and unnecessary withholding of information.
- Detachment – researchers try to remain detached from the phenomenon under study; the wrong approach to do justice to human action.
- Conservatism – research is continually co-opted, and paid for, by those who want to prop up the system, and serves to keep those at the bottom right there.
- Language – research reports are written for the expert in language that mystifies the public, disguising common sense notions.

Research methods which avoid these mistakes are being developed. Feminists have sought to identify and create research methods which, according to Rich (1972) enable Re-vision – the act of looking back, of seeing with fresh eyes, of entering an old text from a new critical direction.

Feminist researchers have questioned the traditional distinctions between subjective and objective, and have emphasized the role of personal experience, of people as their own sources, and the value of studying one's own people. As Calloway (1981) argues, if this is the age of experience in research, as some social scientists have suggested, then perhaps it is the work in women's studies which has helped to create this new emphasis and to make it legitimate.

Action research methods (Hart and Bond, 1995) emphasize getting involved in solving real life problems at the same time as generating new knowledge, learned by doing. Participatory action research stresses that researchers and subjects work together to identify and solve the problem, and that the subjects are involved in decision making about the research and share the new knowledge generated by the research. Both these types of research stem from an understanding that social research does have an effect on the people and situations it studies. This effect should be acknowledged and made conscious, and the subjects of the research given the opportunity to influence and share in the research process and to benefit from it directly. They should be offered the chance to improve their situation and to learn new problem-solving skills. The researcher must be willing to relinquish the unilateral control that the professional researcher has traditionally maintained over the research process (Whyte, 1991).

Existing research on users' views in psychiatry

There is now a growing awareness among mental health workers (both statutory and non-government) of the need to research users' views on mental health services. Much research is being carried out but the extent to which it breaks away from the medical paradigm is variable. However, it is notable that almost any survey of patient or client opinion in mental health reveals a different set of priorities about mental health treatments from those underpinning the biochemical and genetic research which dominates clinical practice. Users tend to rate good human relationships with staff and other patients, listening skills and personal freedom more highly than physical treatments.

Consumer satisfaction surveys of hospitals and treatments

These are often the least paradigm-challenging. Such studies are generally done by mental health professionals or students, with little or no user involvement in planning or carrying them out. They usually contain unstated but pervasive medical or psychological assumptions about the purpose of the research and the population to be studied. One common assumption is likely to be that the patients interviewed are in receipt of medical treatment for their 'mental illness'. If the interviewee believes that s/he has in fact been wrongly imprisoned, assaulted, abused, patronized and lied to, s/he will probably give a defensive or uninformative reply. Many patients will see the interviewer as another psychiatric professional with power over them and will give a reply designed to tell the questioner what s/he seems to want to hear. Maruyama (1974) compared research on prison inmates by outside experts with research done by the prisoners themselves and found that prisoners tended to develop sophisticated methods for giving suitable replies for each different type of professional outsider.

However, even consumer research which does not overtly challenge the medical paradigm can elicit findings which are useful in building a user perspective on the value of medical treatments in psychiatry, as the following examples indicate:

What do psychiatric inpatients really want?
Inpatients in an inner London psychiatric teaching hospital were interviewed about which aspects of their treatment they found most helpful. The most valued item was the freedom to leave, followed by

visitors and talking to doctors and nurses. Drug treatment was judged on average to be only 'quite helpful'. At the bottom of the list came the ward round, talking to other patients and the ward meetings (McIntyre, Farrell and David, 1989).

Patient voices

This study of 62 patients and 25 nurses in Claybury Hospital concerning the items they considered most helpful in acute psychiatric care showed that patients considered having an interested person to talk to more helpful than 'treatment-oriented care', e.g. drugs. Drugs and ward rounds were in the bottom four items. 'Patients are clearly not convinced of the benefits of psychotropic medication.' The patients' responses were remarkably consistent for all the items (Sharma, Carson and Berry, 1992).

Research on users' views carried out by funded voluntary organizations

This kind of research tends to be more user-friendly, and less committed to medical perspectives, though again it varies in how much users have been involved with deciding the questions and in carrying out the research.

Some examples of this kind of research:

Experiencing psychiatry

This was the biggest ever study of mental health service users' views carried out by a voluntary organization. Over 500 service-users answered an extensive survey about their experiences and views of a wide range of psychiatric treatments. General comments were not positive. Many people felt that their views and problems were not listened to. Even more felt that there was an over-reliance on drugs in psychiatry (Rogers, Pilgrim and Lacey, 1993).

The first 24 hours

This is a published report of the process of organizing, and the results of, a public meeting on 'The first 24 hours after admission into a psychiatric hospital'. Attendees were users, relatives and service-providers. Users identified problems such as lack of dignity, loss of control, not knowing where anything is and who are the staff and who are the patients. Suggestions for improvement included better explanations, proper introductions to ward life and personnel, availability of independent advocates, redesign of the hospital environment, more resources for staff and research, and more alternatives to hospitalization such as 24-hour crisis centres (Arnold, Finucane and Rose, 1993).

Users acting as paid or voluntary consultants and researchers for statutory or non-statutory mental health organizations

Two recent examples of this growing genre of user-directed research have been provided by the Sainsbury Centre for Mental Health and the Department of Health's Mental Health Task Force.

The Sainsbury Centre, though not in any sense an anti-medical or politically radical organization, acted on the directive in the NHS and Community Care Act 1990 to involve users and carers in mental health planning. They developed a long-term co-research relationship with a group of psychiatric service users, invited through voluntary mental health organizations such as MIND and established mental health self-advocacy groups. The user group met regularly, with expenses and lunch provided, with workers at the organization, over a period of several years. They acted as consultants to ongoing research into community mental health services, producing their own report, entitled *Whose Service is it Anyway*. They spoke at conferences organized by the Centre, and members of the group were commissioned by the Centre to carry out a user evaluation of a case management project. The Centre provided support in designing and implementing the project and published the final report, while giving final editorial control to the group of three user researchers.

In the report, titled *Have We Got Views For You?*, the researchers set out the case for user-led research:

> It was strongly believed that users, who can demonstrate their common experience with other users, could get at the truth much better because they could persuade others of their independence from the service... In particular, the issue of independence from the service provider is very difficult for non-user researchers. Their background, presentation and links with service agencies make it difficult for users to believe that their views will not get back to those who provide the service directly. They then fear that their service might be withdrawn or that they will be made to suffer for their criticism... The perceptions that [user-led research] seeks are those that users would want to tell each other, not what they have been told is good for them (Beeforth, Conlan and Graley, 1994).

The second example, the Mental Health Task Force User Group, was a large action research project. A group of nine current and former mental health service users, representing the three main user self-advocacy organizations in England, were commissioned to carry out Consumer Satisfaction research during the two-year life of the Mental Health Task Force. The Task Force was an executive group set up by the Department of Health to investigate the closure of the large psychiatric hospitals and the transfer of services to the community. Its main areas of research were good practice in planning and providing new services, financial matters, consumer satisfaction and influencing public attitudes to mental health.

The Task Force User Group, funded and supported by Task Force executive and administrative workers, organized a series of ten regional conferences, a national user conference and five training events for users wanting to be speakers and trainers on mental health issues. A small working group, of whom the author of this chapter was a member, produced a set of guidelines for locally negotiated Users' Charters: a set of nine rights and principles on which users would like services to be based.

These principles were gleaned from research on existing charters of rights and demands drawn up by local and national mental health user groups, and were consulted on very widely through the existing national mental health networks. The results were taken to the national conference, at which 200 users representing local and national groups endorsed it unanimously. The main points of the Charter, reproduced below, represent the aspirations of a large number of psychiatric service users in England. The adoption of these principles would strengthen the users' position in relation to psychiatric experts, leading to substantial change in service provision and stimulating different approaches to research and treatment.

A proposed local charter for users of mental health services

You have the right to:
1 Personal dignity and respect
   be treated with dignity, respect and courtesy at all times;
   privacy and physical safety;
   not to be discriminated against on any grounds.

2 Information
   clear, objective personal and general information in an easily
   understood and accessible form, covering all aspects of your care in
   the mental health services;
   information about your diagnosis.
3 Accessibility
   appropriate services where and when you need them;
   access to community services, such as social services, when in
   residential care.
4 Participation and involvement
   be a full partner in identifying and planning for your own care/service
   needs and drawing up your care plan;
   be present when your needs are assessed and your services planned;
   involvement (at all levels and stages) in planning and development of
   services;
   setting service standards; managing services; monitoring the quality of
   services; and training of staff.
5 Choice
   be offered information about, and receive, a choice of services
   appropriate to
   your expressed (and assessed) needs;
   have your views taken into account if you are not satisfied with your
   keyworker;
   state a preference for a key worker of your own sex.
6 Advocacy
   have someone with you of your own choice, either a friend or trained
   advocate, at any meeting with a professional worker, to provide
   support or to represent you in the way you specify;
   have access to independent advocacy services, in a private setting.
7 Confidentiality and records
   the greatest degree of access to your records allowed by the law;
   to challenge the content of records to which you have access and to
   add your own views;
   to be informed of the confidentiality policy, which will preserve
   confidentiality to the maximum extent that is compatible with
   offering an effective service.
8 Complaints
   have any complaint investigated thoroughly, speedily and impartially,
   and be informed about the progress of a complaint regularly or on
   request;

have information about and access to statutory complaints procedures; not be victimized for making a complaint or your treatment to be adversely affected.
9 Treatment
receive the least restrictive, least harmful treatment that is suitable for you;
be informed of harmful, or potentially harmful, effects of medical treatment;
treatment that is compatible with your beliefs;
be informed of alternatives to medical treatment;
be treated or cared for by a trained, supervised, competent person;
a good standard of medical care, including ready access, whether in hospital or the community, to services such as dentists and opticians (Mental Health Task Force User Group, 1994).

User conferences and consultation groups run by statutory or voluntary organizations or by user groups themselves

These serve several different purposes:
   1 Consciousness-raising, training and education of users, public and mental health workers
   2 Information sharing and networking among users and between users and workers
   3 Giving information about user views to statutory service providers
   4 Challenging the status quo and creating a collective vision and impetus for change
   5 Producing written reports which can be of use in promoting more user-centred services.

The first example of this type of research is a report and manifesto produced following the 1992 Mid-Glamorgan Mental Health Service Users' Conference, an event organized by local users with support from the Mid-Glamorgan Association of Voluntary Organisations and funding from Joint Finance. The report calls for some major changes to services. The Manifesto contains eleven points, of which a few are listed below:

   1 Full involvement in individual care planning and district and county service planning
   2 A range of community services that are regularly monitored (by a

user-led monitoring service) to ensure that quality remains high and that they are provided fairly and equally to individuals across the county

3 A range of crisis intervention services to be developed, including short-term safe houses and places for sanctuary

4 A significant reduction in the use of major and minor tranquillizers and ECT

5 A significant change in the attitudes of staff working in hospitals and a big improvement in the quality and sorts of treatment offered.

One of the key issues raised was that of discrimination against women in psychiatric services as the following quotes illustrate:

- Doctors (often men) contribute to why women feel bad by assuming or implying that the woman's problem or distress has physical causes, such as her appearance, hormones or PMT.
- That a woman's problem or distress is due to neurosis.
- That they know how women feel.
- Male doctors don't or can't listen, so they prescribe drugs.
- Once you have been labelled mentally ill, doctors use it as an excuse not to have to listen to you.

Many of the women who attended the conference had had ECT. They had been told things like, 'It will help you forget the past', if they had been told anything at all. Women were not told about the side effects of ECT (Mid-Glamorgan Association of Voluntary Organisations, 1992).

The second example is the Eating Distress report, produced by Survivors Speak Out, a national mental health self-advocacy organization. This publication was based on a user-run conference held in September 1991 and consists of the speeches given by five presenters. Each one gives a personal insight into the social pressures which lead to eating problems, how it feels to have an eating problem and the frequent insensitivity of psychiatric services to the realities of the patient's life and emotions, as the following quote illustrates:

Whatever way I expressed my distress or dissent it was declared invalid, stupid or sick. The so-called eating disorder label is an inadequate explanation of the very complex reactions and feelings I experience. Indeed for me it is a damaging simplification of an expression of distress which clearly demonstrates the need for cultural and social change... I feel that people labelled as mentally ill experience and express feelings the majority do not allow or open themselves to ... What I am is a woman who discovered at an early age that a woman's worth in our society is based upon her appearance (Pembroke, 1992).

Individual survivor researchers – doing academic or non-academic work, with funding

Two very different examples of this genre are Lindow's (1994) Rowntree-funded study of Self-Help Alternatives to Mental Health Services, and O'Hagan's (1994) report of her study visits to survivor groups in the USA, Britain and the Netherlands.

Lindow, a psychiatric survivor and former chairperson of Survivors Speak Out, describes a number of user-controlled alternatives and the vision needed to sustain such alternatives.

- Judi Chamberlin... stated that self-help alternatives that have only either a support-giving function or a political function are doing only half the job. They need both.
- This civil rights and liberation foundation might be part of a user-controlled alternatives value statement, which could include these and other ideas:
- the equality and value of every individual in the project
- the value of minority opinion, and the freedom to express such views
- tolerance
- optimism about each other
- acceptance of all differences between people that do not interfere with others' rights.

O'Hagan, in her account of the groups she visited, talks about the need for the survivor movement in mental health to link experience with ideology and ideology with practice. She says:

Looking back, this report is the working and reworking of two themes. The first theme can be condensed into the word meaning. What is the meaning of our madness? How does that meaning contribute to the ideology of our movement? The second theme is management. How do we manage our activities so they will truly reflect our ideology? (O'Hagan, 1994).

Both of these reports make their personal and ideological standpoint perfectly clear, and offer their research as a contribution to the movement for survivor-led services. While Lindow writes for a mixed audience of psychiatric survivors, voluntary and statutory service providers, O'Hagan's work appears to be aimed mainly at a readership of psychiatric survivors. However, both have made their work clear, accessible, person-centred and jargon-free, in contrast to orthodox psychiatric research.

Research carried out by individual users without sponsorship or official support

Two examples in this category are the *Users' Report on Psychiatric Services* (Cresswell, 1993) and *The Place of Complementary Therapies in Mental Health – A User's Experiences and Views* (Alexander, 1993).

This first survey was designed and organized by Cresswell, a long-term patient in Broadmoor. It was a remarkable achievement for someone living under such a restrictive regime, and represented an exercise in informal support, cooperation and networking among survivors in hospital and the community.

The survey is open to technical criticisms for some extremely leading questions, e.g. 'users were asked if they believed psychiatric treatment to be a waste of time and public resources', but the results are clearly analysed and the report is of interest not only for its content but also its revelation of the stark division that can exist between between recipients and providers of psychiatric services.

Of the 85 respondents, 50% spoke of treatment side-effects, such as addiction to tranquillizers, and 32% said they had wanted sympathetic counselling which was rarely forthcoming.

The summary of the report states that:

> An overwhelming 76% of people say that psychiatric treatment did not cure them, 5% say there was nothing to cure. Further problems to the ones for which help was originally sought were experienced by over half the users. Despite this, contributors to the survey, for which forms were distributed by mental health organisations, were reluctant to vote for the complete abolition of all mental health services. Whereas 38% of users voted for the abolition of psychiatry, 46% wanted its continuation although many stated there should be more counselling and switching of

funds from hospital to community based services. The suffering of many users under the heading medical treatment is an indictment to [sic] the medical profession (Cresswell, 1993).

Another mental health system survivor, Alexander (1993), a member of Nottingham Advocacy Group, carried out a survey on the benefits of aromatherapy. This survey, though a small sample, is well written up and presented.

Alexander writes about her own experiences with alternative therapies, and reports her interviews with four users who had experienced aromatherapy and reflexology, and a number who had experienced talking treatments.

From her overall conclusions, the following extract is taken:

> The abuse of power personified in the control and management of some individuals coping with a disorientated mind and body are only reinforcing low esteem and adding to their problems. A continuing partnership between Professionals and Users on a more holistic, informed choice and consent basis is indicated by my research. The medication culture must be re-evaluated in the 90s.

These two reports are clear about their own starting point of commitment to user perspectives on psychiatric treatment. Cresswell uses traditional questionnaire methods, with her own anti-psychiatric bias clear from her phrasing of the questions and her analysis of the findings. Alexander makes her personal experience part of the research, and explains both her methodology and its limitations of scope. Cresswell's study is remarkable for her refusal to be silenced, her determination to maintain a network of relationships outside Broadmoor and the support given to her work by user-led organizations. Alexander's study offers a model for user-led research on alternatives to orthodox psychiatric treatment that could be carried out in any small mental health project. The gradual accumulation of such grass-roots evidence could be a major factor in wearing down the edifice of the medical model and normal science in psychiatry.

Conclusions

There are consistent themes in research on user views in psychiatry, regardless of the method of obtaining this information. Survivors or users of psychiatry ask for: more humanity and respect, less medication, more talking treatments, listening, counselling and therapy, more information, more choice of alternative treatments, non-medical asylum or safe-houses, and services which recognize differences in needs based on gender, class, ethnicity or other attributes. These demands challenge psychiatric orthodoxy, which has traditionally emphasized professional boundaries, scientific objectivity, technological solutions to emotional problems, treatments with quick results, standardization of diagnosis and treatment, clinical settings and the central role of the medically-trained psychiatrist.

Survivor or user-led research often overtly challenges the medical paradigm, either subtly or directly in some of the following areas:

1 The concept of crisis or distress is often preferred to the 'mental illness' concept
2 Social or spiritual models of understanding distress rather than medical are proposed
3 Hearing voices and other non-usual experiences are seen as phenomena with a number of possible explanations, rather than as a prime symptom of psychotic illness (Romme and Escher, 1993)
4 Psychiatric treatments are sometimes described as abuse or torture rather than medical treatments
5 medical concepts and language and psychiatric labels are often regarded as damaging, stigmatizing, unhelpful and inappropriate.

Stark differences between survivor-led research and that done by mental health professionals are often revealed in the choice of starting point, subject matter and perspective. While psychiatric researchers generally evaluate existing orthodox psychiatric interventions, from an assumption that mental illness can be clinically defined, survivor-led research often treats the concept of mental illness as open to question. They frequently focus on self-help and alternative treatments.

While orthodox research can result only in recommendations for incremental changes within the existing paradigm, user-led research tends to recommend more radical shifts of control, rights, choices, information and resources to users and user organizations. These changes are not incremental, but discontinuous, requiring a fundamental rethink of the knowledge-base, purposes and control structures of psychiatry. User research indicates the need to replace the dominant biochemical and genetic research paradigms in mental health by complex, holistic research paradigms. Such research would be grounded in participatory action research processes, in which mental health services were continuously evaluated by recipients, some of whom could themselves become researchers and service providers.

The fear and stigma of madness has kept all of society in a straitjacket of normality, which damages our capacity for self-expression, creativity, originality, fun, tolerance and mutual support. A paradigm shift will benefit all but those who profit from the distress and disempowerment of others.

References

Alexander, B. (1993) *The Place of Complementary Therapies in Mental Health – A User's Experiences and Views* (unpublished report). Nottingham Advocacy Group.

Arnold, C., Finucane, J., Rose, N. (1993) *The First 24 Hours*. Manchester: MIND.

Beeforth, M., Conlan, E., Graley, R. (1994) Have We Got Views For You – User Evaluation of Case Management. London: Sainsbury Centre for Mental Health, p. 4.

Blair, P. (1982) Some observations of the cure of mad persons by the fall of water. In *300 Years of Psychiatry* (R. Hunter and I. MacAlpine, eds). New York: Carlisle Publishing. p. 325.

Breggin, P. (1993) *Toxic Psychiatry*. London: Fontana.

Calloway, H. (1981) Women's perspectives: research as re-vision. In *Human Inquiry* (P. Reason and J. Rowan, eds). Chichester: J. Wiley & Sons.

Capra, F. (1983) *The Tao of Physics*. London: Fontana, p. 341.

Cooper, D. (1978) *The Language of Madness*. London: Allen Lane.

Cresswell, J. (1993) Users' report on psychiatric services. *Asylum*, 7, 2.

Harre, R. (1981) The positivist-empiricist approach and its alternative. In *Human Inquiry* (P. Reason and J. Rowan, eds). Chichester: Wiley & Sons, pp. 3–4.

Hart, E., Bond, M. (1995) *Action Research for Health and Social Care*. Buckingham: Open University Press.

Kuhn, T. (1970) *The Structure of Scientific Revolutions*, 2nd edn. Chicago: Chicago University Press.

Laing, R. D. (1970) *The Politics of Experience*. London: Penguin.

Lindow, V. (1994) *Self-Help Alternatives to Mental Health Services*. London: MIND Publications, p. 14.

Maruyama, M. (1974) Endogenous Research vs Experts from Outside. *Futures*, October, 389–394.

McIntyre, K., Farrell, M., David, A. S. (1989) What do psychiatric inpatients really want. *British Medical Journal*, 298, 159–160.

Mental Health Task Force User Group (1994) *Guidelines For a Local Charter for Users of Mental Health Services*. London: NHS Management Executive.

Mid-Glamorgan Association of Voluntary Organisations (1992) *Mid-Glamorgan Mental Health Service Users Conference Moving Forward, Working Together* (unpublished report), pp. 51–52.

O'Hagan, M. (1993) *Stopovers on my way home from Mars*. London: Survivors Speak Out.

Pembroke, L. R. (ed.) (1992) *Eating Distress: Perspectives from Personal Experience*. London: Survivors Speak Out. p. 19.

Peterson, D. (1982) A Mad Person's History of Madness. Pittsburgh: University of Pittsburgh Press, pp. 105–107.

Prigogine, I., Stengers, I. (1984) *Order Out of Chaos*. London: Harper Collins.

Reason, P., Rowan, J. (eds) (1981) *Human Inquiry*. Chichester: Wiley & Sons.

Reiser, S. J. (1978) *Medicine and the Reign of Technology*. Cambridge: Cambridge University Press, p. 227.

Rich, A. (1972) When we dead awaken: writing as re-vision. *College English*, 34, 18.

Rogers, A., Pilgrim, D., Lacey, R. (1993) *Experiencing Psychiatry*. London: MIND/Macmillan, p. 157.

Romme, J. M., Escher, S. (1993) *Accepting Voices – A New Analysis of the Experience of Hearing Voices outside the Illness Model*. London: MIND.

Schon, D. (1971) *Beyond the Stable State*. London: Penguin, p. 216.

Sharma, T., Carson, J., Berry, C. (1992) Patient Voices. *Health Service Journal*, 16 January, 20–21.

Sims, A., Owens, D. (1993) *Psychiatry*, 6th edn. London: Baillière Tindall.

Szasz, T. (1974) *The Myth of Mental Illness*. New York: Harper & Row.

Unzicker, R. (1984) unpublished poem.

Whyte, W. F. (ed.) (1991) *Participatory Action Research*. London: Sage, p. 241.

Chapter 16

Assessing learning outcomes in post-qualifying community care training

Jane Shears, Shula Ramon and Edna Conlon

Introduction

The first multidisciplinary post-qualification course in Britain to focus on continued care clients was set up in 1990 at the London School of Economics. The course, Innovation in Mental Health Work (IMHW), provided advanced tuition for experienced professionals from a health or social services background. It focused on innovation in working with people who are long-term mental health service users, and their carers.

Within the field of education there is a current shift in thinking about how best to evaluate learning outcomes, away from knowledge-based assessments towards performance or competency-based evaluation (Wolf, 1988; Evans, 1990; Black and Wolf, 1991; Powell, 1992). The issue of demonstrating evidence of learning has also begun to permeate social work (Gardiner, 1988; Evans, 1990; McCaugherty, 1991; Girot, 1993). The context of the development of interest in learning outcomes is followed by details about the IMHW course, and an account of the way that assessing learning outcomes for course participants has been attempted.

The conceptual basis for evaluation of practice-based learning outcomes

The fall in the number of traditional apprenticeships, rapid changes and increased sophistication in the field of technology, and increased demands for labour mobility, are all cited by Black and Wolf (1991) as exerting pressure on workers to demonstrate competency in their work practices. These pressures are derived from the managerial ethos, and reflect a move away from a prevalence for academic teaching. Concepts such as occupational competency, accountability, target setting, achieving objectives and developing mission statements, are integral to the developing work ethos in the 1990s.

In the field of social care, the process of training social workers was criticized throughout the 1970s and 1980s, particularly on the discrepancies in the way a student's competency to practise was assessed (Evans, 1990). The Certificate Qualification in Social Work (CQSW) was replaced in 1990 by the Diploma in Social Work. It was intended to address the lack of evidence about a person's competency to practise social work by placing the central emphasis on assessment based on directly observed practice.

The success of these new approaches in the training of social workers is currently being evaluated and updated (CCETSW, 1993; CCETSW, 1994). However, Rushton and Martyn (1993) suggest that the assessment of learning outcomes in post-qualification education, and their application in the work setting, is very rare.

In nursing education too, attention has been turned to the problem of assessing competent clinical practice (Burnard, 1988). The focus of the introduction of the diploma level course in nurse education, Project 2000, is the assessment of students' practice within the workbase setting (Girot, 1993). French (1992) concludes that the UKCC Project 2000 needs to take more account of the importance of the development of practice-based education.

The challenge for the IMHW was not only to bring together workers from different disciplines with different prequalification educational and training experiences, but also to develop more sophisticated ways of assessing course participants' learning outcomes. To reflect the principles of the course, this needed to include ways of involving service users and carers in evaluating the worker's performance, to be non-intrusive, and to take into account that the students are experienced workers as well as adult learners.

Innovation in mental health work – course aims

There are three main aims of the course. The first is to enhance the quality of support to people with long-term mental health needs in the community through the input of new knowledge and skills, and the re-examination of attitudes. The second aim is to enhance the profile of working with this client group for helping professionals. Third, the course aims to demonstrate that this work can be rewarding and interesting, without glossing over the difficulties entailed in the process.

Course components

The duration of the course is 30 days in college (day release) and 30 days of project work undertaken in the student's own workplace. The methods of teaching are designed to make use of the skills and experiences that participants bring to the course as adult learners. Teaching takes place mainly in informal seminars and workshops, enabling participants to discuss and examine their own and others' perspectives of their work. Sessions are organized by five main trainers representing nursing, social work, psychology and psychiatry. Service users and carers, as well as other workers, contribute to the teaching. Course members, too, actively participate in their own learning.

The workbase project requires students to innovate change at their workplace and to involve users or carers in the change process. It enables participants to test the value of their newly-acquired skills and attitudes, and to look creatively for opportunities to develop innovative practice. Examples of projects from course participants in 1993 were: creating a forum for carer consultation about local authority Community Care Plans; introducing a user participation group into a community support unit; developing a local system of crisis cards for service users; and coordinating a support group for single homeless women.

In addition to developing skills in innovation, the course promotes skills in care management, networking, engagement/participation with service users/carers, and counselling with continued care clients.

Course evaluation

Evaluation procedures in place prior to the 1993/1994 intake were focused on written work in the form of two essays and the project report. In 1994, greater emphasis was placed on identifying ways to evaluate learning outcomes in the workplace for the non-project components.

Two new methods of assessment have been incorporated into evaluation or learning outcomes: a personal learning journal and an evaluation questionnaire based on constructs generated from discussions with service users, informal carers and mental health workers. This consultation process reflected the course philosophy of treating service users' and carers' views as equally valid as the workers' views.

Personal learning journal

The personal learning journal is seen as a way for participants to keep track of the events related to the course or work that happen throughout the year, and to relate these events to their thoughts and feelings around them. Students are asked to record one critical event each week, and submit at least one of these events at the end of each term. It provides information from a subjective perspective about what students are taking away from the course and being able to use in their workplace. For example, the National Hearing Voices Network made a presentation on the course based on alternatives to the use of medication. One student discussed the content of this presentation with a service user, and as a result they were able to discuss openly disordered thought processes with the service user. In turn this had led to the workers' greater understanding, and ability to have a more equal and sharing way of working.

The personal learning journals provide a record for the students of the process of participating in the course and also their perceived outcomes of their learning in the workplace. The journals enable students and educators to identify personal progress both in terms of self-assessed newly-acquired knowledge and skills, and also attitudinal changes associated with the experience of the course.

Evaluation questionnaires

A more inter-subjective and participatory attempt to evaluate work-based learning outcomes is the use of evaluation questionnaires. Although the concept of evaluation questionnaires is not new, the difference is that service users and carers, as well as students and line managers, evaluate the students' performance.

Generating the questionnaires

Four established groups of service users and carers were consulted in the London area, including a group of black users and carers. A multi-disciplinary group of mental health workers also participated. Each group was asked to say what they thought the qualities of a good mental health worker (e.g. social worker, care manager, community psychiatric nurse) were. They were also asked the qualities needed to work in partnership with users and carers. From these discussions, twelve qualities emerged:

1 to listen and act on what users and carers say their needs are
2 to be an effective communicator
3 to be a good motivator of others
4 to be flexible and open to change
5 to know the responsibilities of self and others under the Mental Health Act 1983
6 to know the responsibilities of self and others under the NHS and Community Care Act 1990
7 to know how to find and access resources
8 to work effectively with other workers
9 to be committed to working together with service users and other workers
10 to look for the potential in people and situations rather than only the problems
11 to be available to users and carers on their terms
12 to take decisions in consultation with users and carers.

These qualities were generated into constructs and worded accordingly for whoever would be completing the evaluation questionnaire. Each construct was rated on a five-point scale where 1 = Always, 2 = Usually, 3 = Often, 4 = Occasionally and 5 = Never.

The questionnaires were administered in the first term of the course (December, 1993). Course participants, their line manager and a service user or carer with whom the students were working, were required to complete the evaluation questionnaires on three time scales. The time scales were: how they assessed their practice a year ago; how they assessed their current practice; and how they would expect their practice to be in one year's time. The purpose of assessing different time periods was to see what changes in practice and attitudes (as reflected by the course aims) if any, had occurred over time. To assess the longevity of any changes in practice, a follow-up evaluation was planned for one year after students completed the course. Where the line manager was unfamiliar with the student's practice the previous year, another colleague completed the evaluation. As service users or carers had long-term contact with mental health services, they were able to make an assessment of worker's practice the previous year.

Analysing learning outcomes

The data were organized for analysis using repertory grid techniques (Kelly, 1955; Gould, 1991). This method was used because it can accommodate the subjective evaluation of the student's assessment of their own learning, the inter-subjective evaluation of others and the different data sets according to which time frame they represented.

When the questionnaires were returned, only a third of the respondents had completed 'Year from now' forms. There seemed to be some uncertainty about whether these forms should be returned with the others, or next year. Because of this, the 'year from now' data were not included in the analysis.

The response rate for students was 70%, for line managers 63%, and service users/carers 60%. The analysis was conducted using the statistical package SAS (statistical analysis system). Internal consistency was measured using coefficient alpha, with students' ratings measured at 0.75; line managers at 0.72 and users/carers coefficient alpha of 0.83. These results suggested that there was an underlying tendency to rate change consistently across the twelve constructs.

The total change varied from construct to construct. The general tendency was for change in one direction and which corresponded towards perceived better practice. Using the sign test, change was statistically significant in students' rating of themselves for constructs 2, 3, 6 and 9. For line managers, constructs 4, 6, 7, 8, 11 and 12 showed significant overall change. However, for users and carers, significant change was shown on constructs 6 and 7 only. The only consistent construct change as rated by student, line manager and user or carer, construct 6, focused on the workers' responsibilities under the NHS and Community Care Act 1990. This change was perhaps to be expected as students and line managers were grappling with the constraints and opportunities that implementation of legislation was having on their roles and tasks. This may have influenced users and carers, who may have seen changes in the amount and type of resources available to them (e.g. through resources developed with the aid of the Community Care grant, or the Mental Illness Specific Grant). This would appear to be supported by users' and carers' rating of the worker they are involved with as being more able now, than a year ago, to find and access resources.

The users and carers did not rate any significant differences in the constructs relating to attitudinal change. For example, the students gave themselves an improved rating on communicating and motivational skills, and commitment to working together with service users and other workers. However, neither the line manager, service user or carer concurred with these perceived changes in practice. This suggests that although students felt they were acquiring new skills and working in greater partnership with their clients and co-workers, they were not yet demonstrating this in the workplace. As the questionnaire was completed during the first term of the course, there may be some change in rating this construct at a later evaluation.

Line managers' ratings of improved practice tended to focus on workers' adaptability to change, to be more accessible and more effective in their work with other colleagues and in decision making. Although they felt that workers were making themselves more accessible to service users and carers, this was not reflected in how users and carers experienced their contact with workers. This was borne out as no respondents rated any significant changes in constructs 1 and 10 (i.e. that there was no improved rating for students' listening/acting on what users and carers said their needs were, or that users felt that workers looked more for the potential in themselves and their situations, rather than the problems).

As a group of experienced mental health practitioners, it was perhaps to be expected that no changes would be seen to occur in their level of knowledge and understanding of the Mental Health Act 1983. There may be implications for this, however, in terms of refresher training, particularly for Approved Social Workers. Another possible explanation may be that the construct in itself may have been too general to enable any problematic areas from such experienced workers to be highlighted.

Discussion

In attempting to evaluate learning outcomes, the methods needed to be accessible to multidisciplinary practitioners, managers, mental health service users and carers. Furthermore, the aim was to develop evaluative methods which people could use on their own. The methods needed to accommodate both subjective and inter-subjective assessment of the workers' practice, but also produce data suitable for statistical analysis.

The construct questionnaires

Although the alpha coefficient showed rating consistency across the twelve constructs, 'students had a tendency to over-rate themselves. They seemed to rate their practice as, perceived optimum desirable practice', rather than a more realistic assessment of their own practice. One explanation might be that as knowledgeable, skilled and experienced practitioners, they warranted a high rating. They had, after all, been self-motivated in applying to attend the course. The issue of social desirability may also have had an influence on over-rating. It was hoped that these methodological weaknesses could be addressed by asking respondents to rate their practice over time, although a self-serving bias appeared still to be operating.

In terms of presentation, future questionnaires will be structured so that some of the constructs appear as negative. This is an attempt to address ratings from the user and carer perspective. Service users and carers rated improved practice only in the workers' knowledge and understanding of the community care legislation and in their ability to access resources. It is quite possible and indeed more likely that many service users would assess their contact with mental health professionals from a 'less negative' rather than a 'more positive' perspective. For example, recipients of a service may identify with a construct which asks them to rate how often they feel the worker takes decisions on their behalf without consulting them, rather than how often decisions are taken on their behalf with their consultation. It may also be necessary, if this format is to be retained, to revise the way the constructs are worded to take account of comments of specificity and generalizability.

The personal journals

The personal learning journals provided an insight into students' experience of the course and their working environment. Initially the journals recorded concerns and uncertainties in course members' weekly role change from experienced practitioner to student, as they grappled with reconciling two sets of expectations. They negotiated the academic milestones of the first and second essays. The focus of the personal learning extracts changed from a preoccupation with their own role in relation to the course to that of their role as innovator at work. Particular comments stressed the organizational upheavals that seem to feature constantly in many working environments, against which colleagues clung on to established routines, resisting innovative changes in practice. One student described their effort to introduce their innovation project saying that 'some colleagues were not totally receptive to more change as they looked backwards through misty eyes and recalled the hallowed "old order"'. Another student reflected: 'I did not know how much it takes to get people interested in creating change. Keeping the routine seems safe and people do not like to be challenged, but that in the end, I knew it was worth trying. Given the scarcity of knowledge concerning processes of innovation, the personal learning journals have the potential to provide such useful and realistic knowledge'.

Conclusion

'I knew it was worth trying' echoes wider experiences in looking at ways to evaluate learning outcomes. Students clearly valued attending the course away from the pressures at work. They found support from other course members as they attempted to integrate new knowledge and skills into their working environment. Although other colleagues were affected by this process, it had not yet reached service users and carers. This is likely to change for those users and carers who become active participants in the innovation projects.

Ways of evaluating learning outcomes have been developed which give service users and carers an equal share with students and their line managers, in assessing the workers' practice. These results show how important this is to evaluate how successful learning is put into practice. There are some difficulties, but also some strengths in this attempt. This is an example which provides a basis to further the debate, and ways to experiment with new, improved methods to evaluate learning outcomes in post-qualification education.

References

Black, H., Wolf, A. (1991) *Knowledge and Competence. Current Issues in Training and Education.* London: Employment Department Group.

Burnard, P. (1988) Self-evaluation methods in nurse education. *Nurse Education Today*, 8, 229–233.

CCETSW (1993) *CCETSW Review of the Diploma in Social Work*. London: CCETSW Press Release.

CCETSW (1994) *Report of Council Meeting in Glasgow – 21 April 1994*. London: CCETSW Publications.

Evans, D. (1990) *Assessing Students' Competence to Practise*. London: CCETSW.

French, P. (1992) The quality of nurse education in the 1980s. *Journal of Advanced Nursing*, **17**, 619–631.

Gardiner, D. (1988) Improving students' learning – setting the agenda for quality in the 1990s. *Issues in Social Work Education*, **8**, 3–10.

Girot, E. A (1993) Assessment of competence in clinical practice: a phenomenological approach. *Journal of Advanced Nursing*, **18**.

Gould, N. (1991) An evaluation of repertory grid technique in social work education. *Social Work Education*, **10**, 38–49.

Kelly, G. (1955) *The Psychology of Personal Constructs*. New York: Norton.

McCaugherty, D. (1991) The theory–practice gap in nurse education: its causes and possible solutions. Findings from an action research study. *Journal of Advanced Nursing*, **16**, 1055–1061.

Powell, B. (1992) *Measuring Performance in the Education of Adults*. Unit for the Development of Adult Continuing Education.

Rushton, A., Martyn, H. (1993) *Learning for Advanced Practice*. London: CCETSW Paper 31.1.

Wolf, A. (1988) *Assessing Knowledge and Understanding: Methods and Research Priorities for a Competence-based System*. London: Institute of Education, University of London.

Index

References in *italics* are to figures and those in **bold** are to tables

Actual state of healthcare need, 19
Analytical perspective of health, 14–15
Assertive community treatment, 30
Assessment, 33
  learning outcomes, 209–18
    conceptual basis, 209–10
    course aims, 210–15
    discussion, 215–17
  needs, 45–6
    health care, 9–24, 36–7
    mental health patients, 55–72
  skills, 33
Australia, feminist perspectives on
  community care, 99–112
  economic rationalism as masculinist
    discourse, 102
  ideological emphasis on family, 102–3
  long-term strategies, 110
  privatization, 99–100
    dual systems theory, 101–2
    feminist theory, 100–2
    liberal feminism, 100–1
    Marxist feminism, 101
    radical feminism, 101
  short-term strategies, 109–10
  women as care-givers, 103–6
    Australian society, 104
    economic consequences of caring,
      104, **104**–5
    social consequences of caring, 104
    western societies, 103
    women's voluntary welfare labour,
      105–6
  women as clients, 106–9
    Australian society, 106
    lack of understanding of women's
      specificity, 108–9
    structural problems with services,
      107–9

Brief Psychiatric Rating Scale, 63

Brokerage case management model, 30

Camden and Islington Case Management
  Project, 32
Care management, 27–8
Carers, **117**–18
  family as, 117
Caring
  costs of, 118
  economic consequences, 104, **104**–5
  social consequences, 104
  state's role in, 119–20
Case management, 25–42
  definition of, 27–8
  evaluation attempts, 39–40
  evaluative research, 31–3
  interprofessional themes, 37–8
  limits to, 38–9
  needs assessment process, 36–7
  role confusion, 28–9, *30*
  skills, 33–5
    administrative/financial aspects of
      procurement, 34
    assessment, 33
    counselling and psychotherapy, 34–5
    individual service planning, 33–4
    monitoring and evaluation, 35
  social policy context, 26–7
Central Europe, mental health care, 164
Centro al Dragonato, 129–30, 131–2
Change, assessment over time, 62–3
Choice
  benefits of, 49–50
  client, 50–1
  in community care, 90–8
    divided unity, 95–7
    and empowerment, 90–1
    market, 94–5
    and mixed economy of care, 93–4
    self-determination, 92–3
Client choice, benefits of, 49–50

Clinical case management, 30
Communication/cognitive impairment in
    elderly, 73–88
  care recipient as victim of environment,
    75–6
  collection of information, 85–6
  multidimensional approach, 76–85
    environmental context, 83–5
    historical perspective, 76–80
    persons in present, 80–3
Community care
  antinomies of choice in, 89–98
    choice and empowerment, 90–1
    choice and mixed economy of care,
      93–4
    divided unity, 95–7
    market, 94–5
    self-determination, 92–3
  feminist perspectives in Australia,
    99–112
    economic rationalism as masculinist
      discourse, 102
    feminist theory, 100–2
    ideological emphasis on family,
      102–3
    long-term strategies, 110
    privatization, 99–100
    short-term strategies, 109–10
    women as care-givers, 103–6
    women as clients, 106–9
  move from asylum hospitals, 162
Community, as opportunity, 64
Concepts
  health, 14–16
    holistic theory, 15–16
  health care, 16–17
  need, 11–14
    teleological, 12–14
Consumer satisfaction surveys, 196–7
Counselling, 34–5, 142, 147

'Defect' approach, 1
'Deficit' approach, 1
Definitions, 3
Dementia see Elderly, needs assessment
Determination of need, 13
Dual systems theory of privatization,
    101–2

Economic consequences of caring, 104,
    118

Economic rationalism, as masculinist
    discourse, 102
Education, 164
Elderly, needs assessment, 73–88
  care recipient as victim of environment,
    75–6
  collection of information, 85–6
  multidimensional approach, 76–85
    environmental context, 83–5
    historical perspective, 76, 77–80
    persons in present, 80–3
Emotional consequences of caring, 104–5
Empowerment, 90–1
Enabling role, 28–30
Environment
  care recipient as victim of, 75–6
  group, 84
  individual and, 66–9
  personal, 83–4
  physical, 84
European–American perspective, mental
    health care, 161–8
  differences, 164–6
    Central Europe, 164
    USA, 165–6
    Western Europe, 165
  future prospects, 166–7
  similarities, 161–4
    asylum hospitals to community care,
      162
    chronic mental disorder, 162–3
    families, 164
    funding, 163
    homelessness, 161–2
    ideology versus scientific data, 163
    lack of integration, 163–4
    treatments, 163
Evaluation, 35, 39–40
Ex-carers, 120–1

Facilities, MLNA in development of, 49
Family, 164
  as carers, 116
  history of mental health problems, 65–6
  ideological emphasis on, 102–3
Feminist view of community care in
    Australia, 99–112
  economic rationalism as masculinist
    discourse, 102
  feminist theory, 100–2
    dual systems theory, 101–2
    liberal feminism, 100–1

Feminist view of community care in Australia, (cont)
  Marxist feminism, 101
  radical feminism, 101
ideological emphasis on family, 102–3
long-term strategies, 110
privatization, 99–100
short-term strategies, 109–11
women as care-givers, 103–6
  Australian society, 104
  economic consequences of caring, 104
  emotional consequences of caring, 104–5
  social consequences of caring, 104
  western societies, 103
  women's voluntary welfare labour, 105–6
women as clients, 106–9
  Australian society, 106
  lack of understanding of women's specificity, 108–9
  structural problems with services, 107–8
Foundation Sirio, 127–8
Fragmentation of care services, 163–4
Funding, 118, 163
  Central Europe, 164

Gaps in need, 11, 12
Goals
  health, 15, 19–20
  need, 13
Grieving, 146–7
Group environment, 84

Happiness, and health, 15–16
Health
  concept of, 14–16
    holistic theory, 15–16
    and happiness, 15–16
Health care needs
  assessment of, 9–24, 36–7
    concept of health, 14–16
      holistic theory, 15–16
    concepts of need, 11–14
      teleological need, 12–14
    model for, 19–23
  concept of, 16–17
  identification of, 22

object of, 21
population's need for, 22–3
ranking of, 17–19
Holistic care model, 140–50
  basic considerations, 141
  case study, 144–50
  comments on, 143–4
  psychosocial intervention, 141–3
Holistic theory of health, 15–16
Homelessness, 161–2

Identification of health care needs, 22
Implementation paradox, 39
Individual service planning, 33–4
  mental health problems, 63
  use of MLNA in, 47–8
Individual strengths, 63–4
Informal care, Northern Ireland, 113–23
  carers, 116, **117–18**
  context, 113–16
  costs of caring, 118
  ex-carers, 120–1
  State's role, 119–20
Interprofessional relationships, 37–8
Inventory of Socially Supportive Behaviours, 63

Justification of need, 13

Learning outcomes, assessment of, 209–18
  conceptual basis, 209–10
  course aims, 210–15
    course components, 211
    course evaluation, 211–12
    evaluation questionnaires, 212
    generation of questionnaires, 212–15
    personal learning journal, 212
  discussion, 215–17
    construct questionnaires, 216
    personal journals, 216–17
Legislative aspects of care, Switzerland, 124–5
  possible solutions, 135–6
  problems, 132–5
Liberal feminism, 100–1
Life Skills Profile, 63
Local charter, 199–205
  individual survivor researchers, 203–4
  non-funded research, 204–5
  user consultation groups, 201–3

Market, 94–5
Marxist feminism, 101
Mental disorder
  European–American perspective, 161–8
    differences, 164–6
    future prospects, 166–7
    similarities, 161–4
  needs assessment, 55–72
    definition in relation to social access,
      58–9
    disability, access and opportunity, 69
    population, 55–8
    reasons for, 62–3
      assessment of change over time, 62
      planning and design of services,
        62–3
      support and care of individual, 63
    strengths approach, 63–5
    what to access, 65–9
      individual and environment, 66–9
      personal, social work and family
        history, 65–6
      psychiatric service and treatment
        history, 66
Mental health services, Slovenia, 151–60
  contemporary, 153–4
  current, 154–7
  experience, 152–3
  future prospects, 158–60
  history, 152
  overview, 157–8
Methods of needs assessment, 4, 36–7
  mental health settings, 4–6
Mixed economy of care, 93–4
Models
  brokerage case management, 30
  health care needs assessment, 19–21
  holistic care, 140–50
    basic considerations, 141
    case study, 144–50
    comments, 143–4
    psychosocial intervention, 141–3
  needs driven, 61
  service led, 61
Modernization and change, 169–85
  background, 169–70
  change process, 173–83
    consolidation, 180–2
    departures, 182
    irreversible change, 178–80
    planning and preparation, 174–5
    results, 182, **183**
    transition year, 175–8

  goals of reorganization, 173
  implications, 183–5
  information seeking, 170–1
  problems of old organization, 171–3
Monitoring, 35
Multi-level needs assessment (MLNA),
      46–7
  complex cases, 50–2
    matching needs to helper skills, 50–2
  in practice, 47–50
    benefits of client choice, 49–50
    development of facilities and service,
      49
    evaluation of resources, 48–9
    identification of individual need,
      47–8

Needs assessment, 11–14, 36–7, 45–6
  definition of, 44–5
  determination of, 13
  elderly, 73–88
    care recipient as victim of
      environment, 75–6
    collection of information, 85–6
    multidimensional approach, 76,
      77–85
  gaps in, 11, 12
  health care, 9–24, 36–7
    concept of health, 14–16
    concepts of need, 11–14
    model for, 19–23
  integration of care package, 85–6
  mental health problems, 55–72
    definition in relation to social access,
      58–9
    disability, access and opportunity,
      69–70
    population, 55–8
    reasons for assessment, 62–3
    strengths approach, 63–5
    what to assess, 65–9
  multi-level, 46–52
    complex cases, 50–2
    in practice, 47–50
  teleological, 12–14
Needs-based approach, 1–8
  background, 1–2
  definitions, validity and utility, 3
  health care, 16–17
  mental health settings, problems of, 4–6
  needs assessment methods, 4
  other human service fields, 2

Needs-based approach, (cont)
    practical implications, 6–7
New long-stay patients, 56
New long-term patients, 56
Northern Ireland, informal care, 113–23
    carers, 116, 117–18
    context, 113–16
    costs of caring, 118
    ex-carers, 120–1
    State's role, 119–20
Nursing, psychosocial intervention,
        140–50
    basic considerations, 141
    case study, 144–50
    comments on, 143–4
    model for, 141–3

Object of health care need, 21
Old long-stay patients, 55–6

Personal environment, 83–4
Personal history
    mental health problems, 65–6
    relevance to care of elderly, 76–80
Personal learning journal, 212, 216–17
Physical environment, 84
Population need for health care, 22–3
Privatization, 99–100
Procurement
    administrative/financial aspects, 34
    role, 28–30
Programme for Assertive Community
        Treatment, 32–3
Psychiatric service, 66
Psychosocial intervention, 140–50
    basic considerations, 141
    case study, 144–50
    comments on, 143–4
    model for, 141–3
Psychosocial life history, 78
Psychotherapy, 34–5

Quality of Life Interview, 63
Questionnaires
    construct, 216
    evaluation, 212
    generation of, 212–15

Radical feminism, 101

Ranking of health care needs, 17–19
RAWP formula for health care needs
        assessment, 10
REHAB assessment, 62
Rehabilitation service, 43–54
    assessment of needs, 45–6
    definition of needs, 44–5
    future plans, 53–4
    history, 43–4
    MLNA, 46–7
        complex cases, 50–2
        in practice, 47–50
Research
    evaluative, in case management, 31–3
    survivor-led, 186–208
        local charter, 199–201
        novel paradigms, 194–5
        problems of orthodox research,
            186–94
        users' views, 196–9
Resources, evaluation by MLNA, 48–9
Role confusion, 28–9, 30

Self-determination, 92–3
Service
    individual planning, 33–4
        MLNA in, 47–8
    MLNA in development of, 49
    planning and design, 62
    psychiatric, 66
Skills, 33–5
    administrative/financial aspects of
        procurement, 34
    assessment, 33
    counselling and psychotherapy, 34–5
    individual service planning, 33–4
    monitoring and evaluation, 35
Slovenia, mental health services, 151–60
    contemporary, 153–4
    current, 154–7
    experience of, 152–3
    future prospects, 158–60
    history, 152
    overview, 157–8
Social access, definition of needs in
        relation to, 58–9
Social Behaviour Schedule, 63
Social consequences of caring, 104
Social disability, 58
Social history, mental health problems,
        65–6
Social Network Assessment, 63

Social policy context, 26–7
Sociopsychiatric aspects, Switzerland, 124–39
    Centro al Dragonato, 128–9, *130*–1
    Foundation Sirio, 127–8
    future prospects, 136–7
    legislation, 124–5
    legislative/political problems, 132–5
        possible solutions, 135–6
    organizational tendencies, 125, *126*–7
    results, 131–2
State, role in caring, 119–20
Strengths approach, 63–5
Support, 142–3, 148
Survivor-led research, 186–208
    conclusions, 205–7
    local charter, 199–205
        individual survivor researchers, 203–4
        non-funded surveys, 204–5
        user consultation groups, 201–3
    novel paradigms, 194–5
    problems of orthodox methods, 186–94
    users' views, 196–9
        consumer satisfaction surveys, 196–7
        first 24 hours after admission, 197–8
        user-directed research, 198–9
        voluntarily funded studies, 197–8
Switzerland, sociopsychiatric aspects, 124–39
    Centro al Dragonato, 128–9, *130*–1
    Foundation Sirio, 127–8
    future prospects, 136–7
    legislation, 124–5
    legislative/political problems, 132–5
        possible solutions, 135–6
    organizational tendencies, 125, *126*–7
    results, 131–2

Teleological need, 11, 12–14
Tension need, 11, 12

Treatment, 163
    assertive community, 30
    history, 66

USA, mental health care, 165–6
User-directed research, 198–9
Users' views in psychiatry, 196–9
    consumer satisfaction surveys, 196–7
    first 24 hours after admission, 197–8
    user-directed research, 198–9
    voluntarily funded surveys, 197–8
Utility of needs-based approach, 3

Validity of needs-based approach, 3
Voluntarily funded surveys, 197–8

Wakefield Project, 32–3
Western Europe, mental health care, 165
WIPS system, 74
Women
    as care-givers, 103–6
        Australian society, 104
        economic consequences of caring, 104
        emotional consequences of caring, 104–5
        social consequences of caring, 104
        western societies, 103
        women's voluntary welfare labour, 105–6
    as clients, 106–9
        Australian society, 106
        lack of understanding of women's specificity, 108–9
        structural problems with services, 107–8
Work history, mental health problems, 65–6